D0227557

Praise for Yanling Johnson. . .

"Yanling Johnson writes from her own direct experience as a Chinese-born woman and Qigong teacher living with the demands and complexities of contemporary western society. A Woman's Qigong Guide *is an authoritative and valuable guide on the major principles and practices of Qigong and a must read for any woman who seeks to cultivate and benefit from this wisdom in her daily life."*

Gunther M. Weil, Ph.D.
Psychologist, Management Consultant,
Qigong Teacher and Founding Chairman
of the National Qigong Association.

"We are blessed because Yanling had the courage to survive China's cultural revolution and to write this Qigong guide. Her personal story is inspiring, the book well written, clear, informative and essential for any woman trying to live in this stress-filled new millennium. I read it in one sitting and will recommend it to all my clients."

Jeanne Elizabeth Blum
Author: *Woman Heal Thyself*

A Woman's Qigong Guide

Empowerment through Movement, Diet, and Herbs

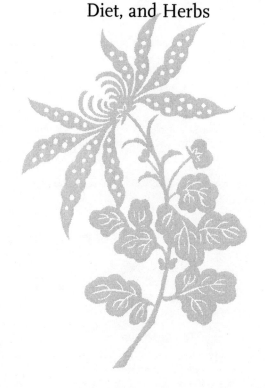

BY YANLING L. JOHNSON

YMAA PUBLICATION CENTER
Boston, Mass. USA

YMAA PUBLICATION CENTER
Main Office: 4354 Washington Street
Boston, Massachusetts, 02131
617-323-7215; ymaa@aol.com
www.ymaa.com

Electronically printed in the United States of America.
November 2002 edition

Copyright ©2001 by Yanling Lee Johnson

Cover design by Richard Rossiter
Text design by Katya Popova

ISBN: 1-886969-83-3

All rights reserved including the right of reproduction in whole
or in part in any form.

Publisher's Cataloging in Publication
(Prepared by Quality Books Inc.)

Johnson, Yanling L.
    A woman's qigong guide : empowerment through
movement, diet, and herbs / by Yanling L. Johnson. —
1st ed.
        p. cm.
    Includes bibliographical references and index.
    LCCN: 00-109784
    ISBN: 1-886969-83-3

    1. Qi gong. 2. Women—Health and hygiene.
I. Title.

RA781.8.J64 2001   613.7148'082
                                     QBI01-200148

Qigong for Women
BY YANLING L. JOHNSON
Health care is public education.
Share my qigong journey and experience.
A book that helps to reveal your own power, to stay healthy and beautiful.

Disclaimer:
The authors and publisher of this material are not responsible in any manner
whatsoever for any injury which may occur through reading or following the
instructions in this manual.
The activities, physical or otherwise, described in this material may be too
strenuous or dangerous for some people, and the reader(s) should consult a
physician before engaging in them.

To all great masters, ancient and modern time
To my late father, my mother, my sister, and brother,
To my children, Claire and Kyle.
To my husband who gave me the opportunity to write

Contents

Foreword

(Translation of 99-year-old Taoist, Zhen Yangzi of the White Cloud Monastery, writing for Yanling Johnson)

AUGUST 18, 1999

"Study abstruse Taoism and its philosophy, practice until attaining Tao and immortalized."

—99-year-old Taoist of the White Cloud Monastery, Zheng Yangzi

Zheng Yangzi is a well-known Taoist who has written several valuable books on qigong and the history of Taoist philosophy. December 14, 1999

The earliest saying of qigong was used by the Yellow Emperor, who consulted his teachers Chi Songzi and Guang Chenzi about Tao and qigong practice. *The Yellow Emperor's Internal Classic* is the first Chinese medical book, which includes a large quantity of qigong practice. The Chinese traditional way for preserving health, anti-aging and healing illnesses has become a rich, profound field. Many high level qigong masters were sages who left us a treasure house of health care. Yanling is helping to share this treasure with the rest of the world.

Li Yu-lin,
Vice Chief Supervisor of the
White Cloud Taoist Monastery

Preface

I wanted to write this book because I feel that it is time to pass on the ancient knowledge of Chinese qigong and philosophy to women of all walks of life. Through the years women have been oppressed by society, and although we have overcome many obstacles, most of us continue to battle for equality.

I remember my mother telling me many years ago that in Shanghai in the 1930s there was a show involving a prostitute who was forced to have sex with a dog. She told me that my father's older cousins took him there. He told her of how terrible it was and how the girl's face was pale and sallow; he never went again. I remember the sadness and slight rage I felt for the girl being so inhumanely treated. I remember meeting women in China who were powerless. These women cared for their extended families and children, only to find themselves divorced and left behind struggling. Their husbands however, went on to hold high government positions.

When I came to the United States, I thought that American men and women enjoyed equal rights and women had the right to make their own choices. Yet, in America, I have met women who feel unfulfilled and are searching more or are continually seeking to improve themselves. I also have met women who have lost their souls in a confused search for freedom. Soon I realized that although American women have struggled long and hard for their freedom and now have more rights than the women do in China, still many American women are abused physically, verbally, and mentally. I understand women from different cultures and different societies still suffer the same conflicts. So, when someone asked me to write a qigong book for women, it seemed apparent that it was, indeed, time to embark on such a task.

I am writing this book with the intent to share with anyone interested, the ancient Chinese wisdom concerning the practice of qigong and cultivation. I have included some of my own experiences with the hope that they will help provide the tools for you to gain self-confidence and to establish balance in your life.

I dedicate this book to the female immortals, to the qigong masters in China, to all my teachers, and to the women of the world.

Much thanks to David Ripianzi who shared my vision for this book and also gave me helpful suggestions and great appreciation to my lovely editor Sharon Rose who worked very hard and put up with my "Chinglish" and stubbornness. Thanks to Dr. Yang and the people of YMAA who have delivered my book to the public.

Chapter 1

*"If one learns but without
thinking, he will be lost;
if one thinks much but without
learning, he will be in danger."*
– Confucius

The History of Qigong
and My Story

Laying a solid foundation is a fundamental part of constructing a building. In this case, the foundation of your new building will be the integration of new habits and ideas that will lead you to a better way of life. This chapter and those that follow will impart to you knowledge that is vital to the successful practice of qigong and cultivation and that will help you to reap the benefits of such internal exercises. It is my wish to share with you the knowledge that has allowed me to live a life that is emotionally and physically balanced.

If you have a basic understanding of the Chinese culture, medicine, and philosophy it will be easier to understand qigong because qigong is rooted in such practices. With that in mind, let us begin our qigong journey with a brief history of qigong.

HISTORY OF QIGONG

The term, qigong, was first used by Taoist Immortal Xu Zhi-yang (A.D. 239–374). There are three main types of qigong in China: Taoist (Daoist), Buddhist, and Confucian. When talking about qigong, Chinese religions often come up because the Chinese monks and Taoists also practice qigong and cultivate as part of their religious practice. However, practicing qigong does not necessarily mean that you are practicing or taking part in that particular religion. It is just that these religions also contain qigong practice. After you read the history, you will understand why.

Taoist qigong originates from Taoism and started approximately 7,000 years ago. Taoism originally was and still is a philosophy; however, a nationalized religion based on this philosophy was recognized about 1,900 years ago. The earliest forms of Taoism, were started by the first six Chinese emperors during the remote period. These individuals taught people how to exercise qi within the body and to adapt to nature. Each were educated and trained by great qigong teachers such as the sage, Peng zu, who was the teacher of the Yellow Emperor. Peng zu was said to have lived for over 1,000 years, while the Yellow Emperor himself lived for over 100 years (Taoism teaches that through qigong practice, human beings can live for a very long time, giving rise to such legends as the life span of Peng zu).

The Taoist philosophy considers the human body to be a small qi field; and nature, including the earth and universe, a large qi field. Thus, balancing qi and compromising with nature to keep healthy and live a long life, such are the main theories that were handed down by those sages.

The first Emperor of China, Shen Nong, taught people how to use herbs to balance qi within their bodies as well as with nature. It is said he was able to scan the qi channels inside the body (I personally know qigong masters that can do this). The original *Herbal Classic*, (*Shen Nong Ben Cao*), was named after him. Even today, the *Herbal Classic* is still one of the most important textbooks for students of Traditional Chinese Medicine (TCM).

The second Emperor, Fu Xi, taught people how to eat foods and to understand spatial relationships of people and places in order to harmonize qi. Feng shui, the theory of how to balance qi in the environment, originated from his theory of *Ba gua*. Based on the Ba gua theory, Ba gua qigong practice, and martial arts (e.g., Ba Gua Palm and Ba Gua Sword) were later created by Taoists.

The fifth Emperor, the Yellow Emperor, taught people to practice qigong and medicine to balance qi. The first medical book, The Yellow Emperor's *Nei Jing* was named in his honor. In this medical book, two-thirds of the content relates to qigong; the remaining text concerns herbs, diet, and diagnosing illness.

Additionally, there are other Taoist texts that were not written by or named in honor of emperors. Two of the most well known are the *I Ching* and the *Tao Te Ching* (*Dao De Jing*). The *Tao Te Ching* is one of the most translated books in history. It was written by Lao Zi who was a great philosopher and qigong master. This book through the centuries has had a powerful influence in qigong and Chinese philosophy. The *I Ching* was written at least 3,700 years ago. The *I Ching* says, "The earth, the universe and human beings are the three in one, the three form one organic whole." In other words, human beings depend on natural resources and compromise with the natural world in order to survive. The *I Ching* is considered the fountainhead of Chinese culture, medicine, and qigong practice. The integration of the *I Ching* with qigong and traditional medical practices gives rise to metaphors such as, "Like the blended water and milk, *I Ching* and medicine are inseparable."

Through the centuries, qigong has developed into many different styles. All of these different styles, however, incorporate the use of herbs and dietary practices because, within the Taoist philosophy, herbs and nutrition are considered to be inseparable from qigong practice for preserving health and prolonging lives. Thus, all Taoists are educated in qigong, herbal medicine, and dietary practices. Many have become experts, achieving mastery through a comprehensive study of the *I Ching*. Following are some of the most famous.

❖ Bian Que, an outstanding physician and a great qigong master (770–476 B.C.), could detect a disease at a very early stage before any symptom was visible. He did this by looking at the facial qi-color of his patients. He taught people to use qigong, foods, and medicine to prevent and relieve pathogenic factors and cleanse the organs. His form, Imitating the Birds and Animals, is still popular today.

❖ Tao Hong-jin (A.D. 452–536) updated the *Herbal Classic* and doubled it in size.

❖ Chen Zang-qi and the King of Medicine, Sun Si-miao, (who both lived during the Tang Dynasty) did additional work updating the *Herbal Classic*.

Over time, other Taoist branches developed their own style that gained popularity during different dynasties. One such branch is the well-known Holistic Zhen Taoist branch (A.D. 960–1279). Its founder was the great master of martial arts and qigong, Immortal Wang Chong-yang. He fostered seven students all whom attained Tao and who later became known as the Seven Immortals. Among the seven were Qiu Chu-ji, Ma Dan-yang, Tan Chu-rui, and female Immortal Sun, Bu-Er.

Qiu Chu-ji, the youngest of the Seven Immortals, established the Dragon Gate Taoist branch that was popular during the Yuan Dynasty (A.D. 1271–1368).

During the Ming Dynasty, the Immortal Zhang San-feng established the Taoist School of taiji and taiji practice became popular. Today, the number of the Taoist religious monasteries that were established based on the philosophy of Taoism still remains small compared with that of the other religions.

During the time that Taoist qigong was popular, Confucian qigong was just beginning to develop. At the age of fifty, Confucius created his style of qigong after he studied the *I Ching*. Confucian qigong has been handed down for generations.

A very important physician and qigong master and Confucian scholar, Li Shi-zhen (1518–1593), spent all his life experimenting and updating the *Herbal Classic* (*Ben Cao*).

Nineteen hundred years ago, Buddhism integrated into the Chinese culture and became deeply entwined with Taoism. Buddhist qigong includes various practices (e.g., Big Cart and the Small Cart) and branches (e.g., Tibetan, Chan). Such qigong practice is recognized in this quote from Lord Buddha: "If one only limits self in practicing the Small Cart without merging the Big Cart practice, it will be like burned seeds or spoiled sprouts."

The Buddhist *chan* practice, (*zen* in Japanese) was brought to China in the year of A.D. 527 by the 28th successor of the Lord Buddha, Damo. He taught chan practice at the Shaolin Temple in Henan Province where self-defense type of martial arts had been passed down since about A.D. 500.

Throughout history, the philosophies of Buddhism, Taoism, and Confucianism began to integrate as they all shared a commonality: the idea of individual effort in compromising and harmonizing with nature. Because of this commonality, Buddhist, Taoist, and Confucian qigong were able to co-exist and yet retain their individual identities.

I have read ancient qigong books written by Taoists who also included Buddhist qigong practices and vice versa. Chinese classic literature often contains stories of martial arts masters (Taoist qigong masters and Buddhist monk qigong masters alike) who were traveling together and teaching each other. A well-known Buddhist qigong master who was also a Confucian scholar, Fu Jushi (A.D. 420–589), wore a Taoist cap, a monk's coat and a pair of Confucian scholar shoes to show people the integration of the different schools of thought and the many types of qigong.

Great masters made few distinctions between philosophical schools of thought, religions, or kinds of qigong practiced. When such masters attained a high level of understanding, it was realized that there were no differences. Think of it as building many different roads to the same city.

Such integration of knowledge and practice has made it possible for qigong to integrate with health and general healing and develop into a systematic, comprehensive, and profound field. According to the research of Dr. Liu Tian-jun, there are about 2,700 types of qigong today; 80% Taoist, 10% Buddhist, the remainder are Confucian and folk styles.

The practice of qigong has endured much through the centuries. Some masters tried to develop qigong practice into religions; others—such as politicians like Mao Zedong—oppressed qigong for personal gain. Yet qigong always stays true to its origin and always perseveres. Qigong has been full of vitality for at least 5,000 years and has never been controlled by an individual—and it never will be.

Qigong has been a Chinese treasure for thousands of years to both men and women alike. Even Emperor Qin Shi Huang (221–207 B.C.) would not burn any medical, qigong, or diet books even when he ordered all the books that he could find be burned (and more than 200 well-known scholars to be buried alive). Qigong has been kept alive in the Chinese culture through word of mouth and through the books written by masters from ancient times to present day. Such books have been preserved for centuries by individuals, emperors, and kings, as well as in the temples. Until recently, much of this treasure has been kept from the rest of the world primarily because of language differences and politics: the Chinese language is not easily translated into other languages, and, until recently, political tensions have made such texts difficult to obtain. (Recently, political relations have eased up enough to allow ancient texts to be more accessible to those that can translate them.) At last, it is possible for eastern ideas and philosophies to be brought to the people of the west.

You will see in the following chapters that qigong practice closely entwines itself with dietary practice and herbal medicine. Because qigong is a self-effort to balance and conform oneself to nature, the practice is always based on the individual practitioners needs, will, and consciousness. Thus, qigong becomes a form of self-education not only in its practice, but in eating habits and herbal formulas as well. I like to think of it as a three-in-one healthcare system.

EASTERN HEALTHCARE PRACTICES

Having lived in the United States for fifteen years, I have had the opportunity to become familiar with western healthcare, and I have noticed considerable differences between eastern and western healthcare systems. In order to help you better understand qigong, let us look at how qigong healthcare compares to western healthcare.

1. The primary focus of western healthcare is to take care of an individual after he or she has become ill. In the Chinese culture, prevention of illness is more actively stressed as the first priority. Qigong plays an important role in this prevention strategy. The philosophy of preventive healthcare was evident in the Chinese culture 5,000 years ago. An ancient teaching by the Yellow Emperor states, "To eat and exercise to prevent is more important than to heal. A good physician will treat an illness before it happens."

Building up such inner strength is the root of qigong practice.

2. In the west, building muscle mass through resistance training and intense physical exercise is a popular way to keep fit. According to Chinese health theory, too much exercise can be just as harmful as too little exercise. Therefore, building the outer structure in excess does little for inner cultivation. Only the appropriate amount of physical exercise will yield the most benefit; thus, proper balance must be found. Qigong exercise *cannot* only take care of inner healing, it can take care of the physical body as well.

3. The Chinese mainly seek healthcare through natural sources. I do not find much of this practice in western medicine. I have observed that western medicine depends a lot on modern technology and synthetic chemicals.

4. Western medicine treats eating disorders, anxiety, obesity, hypertension, etc. as diseases. To Chinese medicine these are only symptoms and not the cause or root of the problem. According to the Yellow Emperor's *Nei Jing*, disease is described as follows: "When a symptom shows, the illness inside the body has been there for a long time."

5. In Chinese medical theory, the qi channels that exist in the body can decide a person's health condition, life, or death. In order to experience optimum health, these channels must exist in an unblocked state or illness will occur. It is also believed that emotions are a major cause of most illnesses because they affect the circulation of qi. For example, when cancer is being treated with traditional Chinese medicine, the doctor will focus on both removing the blood stagnation in the patient by promoting qi circulation and treating the patient's emotional state.

Thus, you can see why from the Chinese perspective, in order to get to the root of a problem it is necessary for the integration of qigong practice, herbal medicine, and diet. This integration works on strengthening the qi within our bodies. Learning to integrate these three sciences is known as *cultivation*.

This book will take you on a journey of understanding cultivation. This journey will teach you qigong practices that have been designed to especially benefit women. At the same time, you will journey into the realm of fundamental Chinese philosophies and the principles of traditional Chinese herbal medicine and dietary practices. Since all of these disciplines are entwined, you will get a good idea of the qigong way so that you can add balance and harmony to your life.

WHY QIGONG FOR WOMEN?

Women are built differently from men, both physically and mentally, so it makes sense that there are qigong practices specific for each sex. Specific rules concerning qigong practice that differ from men are highlighted throughout the text. Certainly Chinese philosophies and medicine apply to both men and women, and, of course, both men and women practice qigong, but qigong addresses the differences as well as the similarities. In the *I Ching*, men and women share importance and are compared to "the heaven and the earth"; yet the *I Ching* also shows their differences and compares such differences to "water and fire." Unfortunately, China was and still is a male-dominated society, so most of the time the ancient texts that were written focused on the needs of males. Because there are not many qigong books for women, it is from my heart that I wish to share these treasures with you. I would like to remind women of all cultures to be aware of their inner power and to know the potential that they possess but have not yet explored. The exercises found in this book can teach you to absorb energy from the universe in order to prevent illness, create a healthier physical and emotional life, and promote spiritual growth. I sincerely believe that qigong practice helps put you in touch with yourself—physically, emotionally, and spiritually.

In many cultures, women are often linked to flowers, and I think it is good to be identified with such beauty. If your goal is to preserve health and beauty, learn the theory behind qigong, practice persistently, and your goal will be achieved. Qigong practice can bring out your most valuable qualities. Qigong can help you become your own person in touch with the universe. The first step toward this goal is to study the theory. Such study will prepare your mind and body. Once you are ready, the next step is to bring out your own being.

Within this text I have translated and include in this text a few partial Chinese poems written by various ancient sages. The one you are about to read is about happiness, a state that I feel we all desire on one level or another and a state that, with the proper cultivation, will be more attainable to you. I hope that you enjoy the poems. When you read them you can replace *he* with *she*. The best way to understand them is to read them repeatedly and reflect on their meanings.

> He or she *who knows how to be happy avoids trouble instead of*
> *stirring up trouble.*
> *He who knows how to be happy turns big problems into small ones.*
> *He who knows how to be a happy person turns small*
> *trouble into none.*
> *Avoid talking too much after drinking,*
> *Avoid getting upset when eating,*
> *Learn to tolerate the things that are very difficult to tolerate,*
> *And do not argue with an unreasonable person.*
> *One gets sick only when they eat without control,*
> *And when they constantly worry, death is waiting for them.*
> *Tolerance is the treasure of the xin (heart-mind),*
> *Intolerance is the root of trouble.*
> *The tongue stays long in the mouth because of its softness;*
> *The tooth is broken because of its hardness.*
> *Think of the tolerance as a recipe for happiness.*
> *Those who cannot be tolerant for one minute*
> *Will only live a long, miserable life.*
> *Money is the root of trouble,*
> *To make money is only for building up a business.*

Money is the root of anxiety,
Which can also cause all kinds of trouble.
If one does not love money,
That will be the start of attaining Tao.
One who pursues Tao forgets the shape of their body;
One who cares about health does not indulge in gains,
One who has attained Tao forgets their xin (mind/heart).
I enjoy living carefree although being poor;
And climbing up the mountains to see the scenery, and resting under
*   the big tree,*
I bathe in the springs, and I collect the food fresh.
I enjoy the delicious food from the mountains,
And the delicious fish from the stream.
I get up whenever I like, which is my leisure.
I do not seek fame; that only lasts temporarily,
And rather not leave praise or blame when I am gone.
Who would like to have worries later,
Although he seems now enjoying the gay?

– Han Tui-zhi

THE BUDDHA WITHIN

There is a Chinese saying, "Everyone is born a Buddha." Essentially, this means that we are all born with emotional, physical, and spiritual clarity. Unfortunately life's hardships and corruption can bury the Buddha deep inside us. Yet, through qigong practice and cultivation, your Buddha can be released. In other words, qigong practice can put you back in touch with your inner self.

Some time ago, I was watching a television special on the life and teachings of Jesus Christ. This program brought to my attention one of his teachings that he shared with his disciples. He told them, "If you want to know who I am, you must first know yourself." To me, this great sage was saying the same thing as finding the inner Buddha or the real being inside. Many such ideas can be found in the teachings of Buddhism, Taoism, and Confucianism as well.

Imagine feeling in control of yourself and at peace! As you learn and practice qigong, you will become aware of and be able to experience some of your own internal power. The more you practice, the more aware of your internal power you will become. By using your own internal power, you will become healthier, feel alive and vital, and—frankly—look younger naturally. (Most qigong practitioners look and feel younger than before they practiced qigong. I have never spent money on expensive lotions. I look younger because of my qigong practice). This book is designed to start you at the beginning and lead you through a journey of knowledge and self-actualization. If you work at it, you really can awaken the Buddha within you.

Educating yourself, believing in yourself, and allowing yourself to use your own wisdom to make decisions is to understand the true spirit of qigong. It is my intent that you will learn how to teach yourself to listen to and trust your instincts. Arm yourself with knowledge because with knowledge comes self-control and confidence. For example, after reading this book, you may seek out a teacher and good books to help you on your journey. When you have a good foundation of knowledge, you will be able to recognize unqualified teachers. I have seen some qigong teachers or healers that do not know much about qigong theory at all. Many have not practiced enough to gain the ability and experience to teach or treat you. You need to be sure that what someone is trying to teach you, is, in fact, the real thing and not something that they know little about. Great qigong masters carry the sentiment, "To give the readers wrong information would be worse than murdering." My point is that to believe blindly and only depend on the help of another is not real qigong practice. You must strive to educate yourself and practice persistently.

I hope my story and this book can help you understand what qigong really is and why cultivation is crucial to qigong practice so that you can begin your qigong journey headed in the right direction.

MY STORY

My story will show you how I have been working on my emotions and how I learned to deal with my problems and face the real world by studying the teachings and wisdom of many classic books—including many about qigong. Frankly, I was not aware that it was qigong theory; these principles within Taoism guided me in my young life and helped me to find compromise, balance, and harmony in my life. I have always followed these principles. There have been times in my life—and I am sure there will be more times to come—that my qigong practice and cultivation has helped me grow to the next level of my existence.

Please allow me to share with you briefly some of my life so that perhaps it can in some way be helpful in your life. Although I have suffered many setbacks and disappointments in my life thus far (and who has not?), I have been able to remove bitterness and anger from my heart and replace it with forgiveness. I simply learned to turn my attention to the future. My qigong practice and cultivation has done this for me, and this is why I share this gift with you.

I was born in Beijing, China, the third daughter of a judge and general of the pre-nationalists, as they were called. It was the nationalist government that was overthrown by Chairman Mao Zedong's communist government. Many nationalists fled to Taiwan. Some, like my father, stayed because Mao's government promised him that he could keep his job if he helped them. But eight months later he was put in prison without a trial after the communists no longer needed his help.

As a child I had many varied ambitions as I grew up. I had many opportunities to watch martial arts and qigong performances and so, as a young child, I wanted to be a martial arts master to save the poor and punish evil. When I entered the third grade, I became interested in being a writer, and before graduating from junior high, I wanted to be a vocal soloist. I experienced many activities like singing in the choir for high school girls and playing on the district basketball team.

All in all, I was a typical child with many ambitions and dreams—but at that time in China, it was politics and government that decided your fate. The government did not trust the families of former nationalists and watched us very closely. Many of us did not know that we were distrusted. We were told that as long as we loved the communist party and worked hard, we would all be treated as equals. This is what I believed.

When I graduated from junior high school, I could not go to the music school because the school was closed during the three famine years. I chose instead to go a boarding high school, the Beijing Foreign Languages High School. I chose English as my major and had dreams of being a journalist or a radio host to foreign countries. I enjoyed being chosen to be the lead roles in the foreign language festivals each year and was the school radio broadcaster for a half year; yet later I was dismissed because I was the daughter of a former nationalist.

My family's former political background removed me from ever fitting into any popular girls' groups during my seventeen years in school. Young students my own age were taught that all children of former nationalists were influenced by their parents and should be watched and reeducated. No one wanted trouble, so the other students shunned me. I learned not to fit in from a young age. The many classic books that I read taught me not to care much about popularity. I occupied myself with books and other activities, and I had teachers that cared about me and helped to guide me. I considered myself "a crane standing among chickens," i.e., standing head and shoulders above others, and I was proud of my achievements. I took any unfair political treatment to me, as a personal test and I believed that good would indeed be rewarded.

The government and school authorities taught children like me that their families were criminals of the government. They said that all rich people like my father had the blood of innocent people on their hands and in order to make amends for what he had done I had to become a different person than my father. So, I brainwashed myself by reading Mao's boring books and followed his teachings: "Serve the people and the Party with one heart. Be honest and loyal to the Party." I believed in Mao's book ("The Little Red Book"); I believed that the Party and Chairman Mao did not mean to treat people unfairly, and I was optimistic and hopeful about my future. I wanted to go to the college of my dreams.

I graduated from high school as planned. Yet, even though I did quite well in the entrance examination, the government sent me to an ordinary college because of my father's politics. Students that had much lower grades but that were politically qualified were sent to the best universities. My former classmates told me in later years that there were files kept on rich families and the families of former nationalists that were stamped, "Only allowed to go to an ordinary college."

I was angry and quite disappointed. After some time, I put to use what I had learned and calmed down. I put aside negativity and looked for the fortunate side of the situation. It was extremely difficult for students who were from families like mine to get any chance at all to attend college and, although it was not my ideal choice, it was a chance to attend college nonetheless.

I still studied hard and was a good student, but I no longer had career dreams. I became increasingly more silent. I sang often to soothe my depression. I joined the ice skating team, skating in endless circles to forget the real world. Most of my spare time was spent in the library. Reading was not just a hobby; it was a way to escape and forget. Early in the summer of 1966, terror suddenly enveloped Beijing; the Cultural Revolution began and changed the lives of millions of Chinese people. This happened because of Mao's failed economic policies, causing his supporters among his colleagues to loose faith in him. Knowing this Mao staged a mass political movement that became known as the Cultural Revolution. Mao called on young high school students to start this movement so that he could dispose of those that disagreed with his ideas. He directed these students to establish Red Guard organizations that replaced those government authorities that did not carry out his policies. This movement spread like wildfire in high schools and junior high schools and then into colleges and elementary schools. The Red Guards were encouraged to travel throughout the country to promote this movement. They punished anyone that they thought was not loyal to Chairman Mao. Former landowners, former nationalist officials and officers, former capitalists, anyone who opposed any of Mao's policies was whipped, beaten, jailed, or killed. Over twenty million people lost their lives.

Most young people participated non-violently in this movement, in fact, but took advantage of the situation to travel. I, too, wanted to travel, but I dared not go alone because of my family situation; I joined a team led by a Red Guard member that believed in non-violence. He was leading a long march to go to the early revolution base in Yanan County. On foot, I walked for over a month with my teammates to get there. We stayed in Yanan County for a week before taking a train to the south of China. It was during this trip that I saw the poverty in most of the countryside and realized that politics and hunger for power was covered by beautiful promises. My last bit of hope for the communists and Mao was torn to pieces. For the first time in my life, I opened my eyes to what politics had done to my country and my life. Just before we traveled to the south, my team was called back to Beijing. About eight months later, all of Mao's enemies had been removed and the young students were no longer needed. Mao's trusted PLA took over the schools and the students, including the all the Red Guards, were called on to begin their studies. Four years later, I graduated from college and became a high school teacher, living a quiet life so as not to draw government attention to me. Still, I kept the teachings from the classic books in my mind. They reminded me to live with integrity and decency. I was no longer interested in politics.

I married a young engineer and after a year and a half, our lovely, bright little girl added colors to my pale life. I offered the best education to my little daughter and hoped that she would have a chance to fulfill her dreams. Unfortunately, I married an unfaithful husband who would not stop cheating. I stayed with him because, despite his infidelities, he was a loving father that I did not want to take him away from my child. We had a second child together—my loving son—but still the cheating continued. Divorce was not easy in China, so I stayed in that marriage for fourteen years. I buried my own dreams deeply in my heart and lived mainly for my children and their education. I managed to fit daily qigong practice into my life, and I honestly believe it was qigong that helped me maintain a balanced emotional state during such difficult times. As you can see, my cultivation taught me to forget and tolerate. Being able to do so is a positive power that can induce the *yang qi*—the energy that is light and that benefits health. This was the reason that I did not often feel a heavy heart and avoided falling into the hole of depression.

When China finally opened its door to the west, a small number of scholars were given the opportunity to come to the United States. In 1985, I came to graduate school in Oregon. In the end, I did finally get a divorce.

When I arrived in America, feeling free was an unspeakable joy. Being able to move about freely without a permit from the police station was a freedom that I had never enjoyed. Very soon, I learned to speak freely and without my habitual caution. However, I did not let this freedom overwhelm me. My past experiences and the balance that qigong added to my life gave me the power to keep my mind clear and focused. I let go of my ex-husband, but I still was concerned for the children I had left in the care of their father in China. My heart was like the mother's heart in the following 1,700-year-old poem:

The loving mother is stitching,
Holding a needle with thread.
Stitching, stitching, she sews, and the thread is extending,
As if it were connecting the coat
On her son who is travelling,
A thousand miles away.
No matter how far he travels,
His mother's caring thoughts
Are like the thread in the needle
Extending, extending in her hand and,
So she sews, and sews
For him day after day
As if the thread is connecting
Herself with her son
On his journey to accompany him.

I was trying to find a new life for my children and myself. During this time of change, my qigong practice helped ease my concerns, gave me comfort and stability, and taught me more of the spirit of tolerance and forgiveness.

As I started to interact with the women in this country, I began to see what my culture had given me; my cultivation and qigong practice had empowered me. I discovered that many American women were trapped in lives of emotional imbalance. Some had marriage problems or suffered physical and mental abuses from their spouses; others were divorced and raising small children as single parents. Many had problems with their own parents, families, and inlaws. Others had become confused about life and had difficulty dealing with reality, especially trying to exist in a highly competitive and materialistic society. Having to live with such situations every day, it is easy for us to lose a connection to ourselves. If you exist in a state of emotional imbalance caused by social trappings or undue stress, you then open the door for physical ailments to follow.

WOMEN IN CHINESE QIGONG HISTORY

Although my culture is different, we still have a common bond: we are women. Just like American women, Chinese women have struggled through oppression and are now taking new roles in society—roles other than that of wife and mother. Chinese culture has taught them to be humble and hardworking professionals in a wide variety of fields, including education, science, and medicine to name a few. Many Chinese women practice qigong and have become masters at high levels.

Throughout Chinese history, there have been many women who have made their marks in qigong history. Additionally, there have been famous female poets, gifted scholars, generals, and physicians, as well as many well-known female masters of qigong, martial arts, and the *I Ching*. A few of them are mentioned below.

❖ Some females have been recognized as immortals and spiritual leaders, such as Madame Wei Tsun-hua (Jin Dynasty, A.D. 265–420). Madame Wei was the founder of an important Taoist branch at the Mountain Mao Monastery. Her book, *Huang Ting Classic*, is one of the most important books on qigong. It contains information such as formulas for preparing a qigong practitioner's body for higher level practice. Madame Wei was a high official's daughter; she was very erudite and also an expert at making longevity formulas. According to legend, she left our planet by "stepping on her sword, suddenly flying up, and disappearing at the age of 87."

❖ (As mentioned earlier) the female Immortal Sun, Bu-er (Song Dynasty, A.D. 960–1279) was also a Taoist leader. Immortal Sun assisted her husband, Immortal Ma Chong-Yang, in establishing the Taoist House in their home and financially helped five other Taoists who all were the disciples of Immortal Wang. (These seven became the famous Seven Immortals who all attained Tao and contributed much knowledge to qigong history. Immortal Sun was one of the first Immortals to attain Tao among the seven. Their statues are still worshiped today in the White Clouds Monastery in Beijing.

❖ Of course, you have heard the story of the martial artist, Mu-Lan. Mu-lan learned martial arts from her father at a young age. She then joined the army disguised as a man to fight in place of her father. Her story is still popular in China today and is told in various operas.

I have named but a few of the famous women from China's ancient history but many more exist. There are more female immortals whose names will be mentioned in the poems that I have translated and included throughout this book. It is my hope that, through cultivation and qigong, we will strengthen our physical and mental conditions and that more women can rise above adversity and perform to their fullest potential just as these women have done.

In China, there are thousands of ancient books written by sages who preserved their health and lengthened their life spans. In their texts they share with us how they preserved their lives and how they revealed their inner beings. During my ten years of research and study of qigong and my many years of practicing it, I have learned that, in many ways, we are all the same regardless of race, culture, religion, or age. We all possess internal powers that can be brought out by qigong practice. Such human potential can be cultivated and used to prevent illness, heal an illness that has already occurred, develop the confidence to overcome obstacles and form harmonious relationships with others. The list of what can be accomplished by revealing such potential is virtually limitless. The methodologies that develop human potential for health prevention, however, are still an open question to modern science.

Because of its long-lasting qigong culture, China is a gold mine of natural healthcare methodologies. However, one can only grow by understanding this culture. Whoever sets her (or his) mind on digging will find the gold and become "wealthy."

Chapter 2

Qi and Qigong

Recently I found a book co-written by Chinese medical doctors and researchers. It includes 1,278 cases of patients suffering from various kinds of internal ulcers. These patients all received qi treatment from masters. They also practiced qigong during the course of their treatments. The rate of curing success was greater than eighty percent. Why did this qigong treatment work successfully? The answer is that qigong exercise can regulate the unbalanced function of the cerebral cortex and central nervous system of the cerebrum, which is the cause of ulcers according to traditional Chinese medicine. I know that if you have never been exposed to the concept of *qi* and *qigong* theory, this possibility may seem a little abstract. But as you begin to learn more about qigong theory you will come across concepts that will help to solidify your understanding. As I have mentioned earlier, in western medicine it is common practice to treat the illness or injury after it has occurred. According to Chinese medical thought it is better to prevent the illness or injury from happening at all. This happens by keeping you body and mind in balance through qigong practice and cultivation. The information in this chapter is intended to provide you with a basic knowledge of the general concepts associated with qi and qigong practice.

WHAT IS QI?

Qi energy can neither be created nor destroyed, but it can be stored. Though it may seem mystical, it is really not. Take electricity for example. Electricity is an energy that remains invisible to the human eye, even though we know that it exists. Only when we can physically see the result of electrical current, like a light going on, do we fully appreciate this invisible energy. Qi is very much the same. Unlike electricity, however, the existence of qi has not yet been proven by western science. Qi is not only the sole source of all living things, but it is also spiritually and directly related to our minds. Qi is considered the "commander of the blood," meaning that when qi moves, the blood circulates; if qi movement is stopped then the blood movement also stops. For example, if a sudden injury causes a qi blockage to occur, the blood will not move either and a stagnation like a bruise will occur. Therefore, if the commander (qi) is not in good shape, then the troops (the blood) will not be in good shape either. A common Chinese saying is "When the mind is at ease, the qi will be in harmony." A person's emotional disturbances as well as physical maladies can cause qi blockages, and the qi blockages can lead to health problems and even death.

A friend of mine said, "qi is unnameable." This is true. The word, qi, is a word that seems to transcend definition going beyond words into the realm of experience. Qi is defined as the basis of life. According to Chinese culture, all living things require qi; in Western terms, qi is defined as vital energy. Qi theory is a cosmic theory that is originated from the Ba gua theory and the *I Ching*. Its philosophy includes medicine, diet, qigong exercise, biology, psychology, sociology, astronomy, chemistry, geography, astrophysics, humanities, and anatomy. The qi theory states that because human beings and all living things on our planet were produced from the qi in the universe, so each part of the human body is related to the movements in the universe. The Taoist symbol of yin and yang vividly depicts the movement of all things in the universe, from the energy within our own bodies to the expanses of the solar system. (Figure 1: Yin and Yang) In fact, this cosmic theory is not only found in the Chinese culture. For example, in the Mayan culture, there are Galactic Seasons, the Galactic Core, and Solar Plexus that all relate to nature and the movements of the stars in the universe. Such theories permeate cultures worldwide.

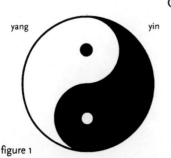

yang   yin

figure 1

The book, *I Ching and the Eastern Nutritology* (written by Dr. Xie a senior researcher and doctor of traditional Chinese medicine) includes a 1984 experiment involving qigong masters. At the Chinese Space Medicare Research Center, the brains of the qigong masters were studied as they meditated. The resulting photos of their brainwave patterns showed a vague picture of the yin and yang pattern. It was also observed that when the masters reached a deep meditative state, their qi penetrated deep into their body tissue right at the places where the main qi channels are. Such results can be reproduced only when every part of the body is in absolute balance.

In order to explain how important qi is to our body, I have translated different explanations concerning qi from various Taoist classic books. One Taoist (name unknown) described in his book,

"When a person has plenty of qi, *he or she* is alive; when the qi dies out, the person dies; when the qi inside is strong, the person will be physically strong; when the qi becomes weak, the person becomes physically old."

The *Shi-Yi* (the book that originated the *I Ching*) in the chapter of Xi Ci says,

> The qi channels resolve life and death and is a crucial factor of healthy and any illness, so they must not be blocked. A good doctor will prescribe according to the qi changing in the seasons, the changes of the weather, the geography, and the individual.

The Taoist metaphoric term for qi in the universe is "mother," and the qi with which a person is born with is "fetus." Thus, through Taoist philosophy we understand that if the fetus is away from the mother, the fetus will die. Only when the fetus is nourished by its own mother will the fetus grow. A well-known Taoist, Ge Hong (A.D. 284–363), whose family was considered a living qigong history and had a powerful influence in making longevity formulas, described how qi can prolong lives and can be formed into *dan*. (Dan is a Taoist term for the longevity medicine that a qigong practitioner produces and delivers by him/herself.)

> After the clam absorbs qi for a long time, a pearl is formed; when a rock absorbs it for a long time, jade is produced; when a human being absorbs it for a long time, the dan will be produced.

The qi theory comes from the word, Tao, which can be found in the *I Ching*. There are no suitable words to define Tao. Let us say that it simply means "the Way." It is not a set of rules; it is not a destination. It is a journey, more or less, through life based on harmony in nature. It is a philosophy and a lifestyle. For an individual qigong practitioner, following Tao specifically nourishes the primary qi with which she (or he) is born. When the qi inside the body is not protected but consumed, it affects the three treasures of the body called *jing, qi,* and *shen.* These three treasures represent qi in motion. When we start cultivating and tapping into our qi sources, they take on these specific properties.

❖ Jing is defined as essence or the source of your body's qi.

❖ Qi is also called post-birth qi. It is your internal energy—your vigor.

❖ Shen is your spirit—the part of you that you are always seeking to enlighten. Shen is the concept that leads the practitioner of qigong down the path to good and balanced physical and emotional well-being.

The following ancient writings explain qi. Please read them repeatedly so that you can have a better understanding. The word, *dan,* is defined above; *tian* translates as "field." The lower, middle, and upper dan tian play different roles; step-by-step they can help qigong practitioners make progress in their practice (see Figure 2). If your interest lies in healing, the lower dan tian is more important. Cultivating qi in the lower dan tian also builds the foundation for advanced practice. To show you how the three dan tian work, I have translated an explanation of an ancient high-level qigong master (name unknown).

"The lower dan tian (which houses the qi with which you are born) is for storing the qi until there is plenty, so that one day, it can move up to the Ni Wan Palace (the upper dan tian). This is called returning the jing that tonifies the brain. If you want to nourish your shen, you have to nourish the qi first; if you want to nourish the qi, you have to nourish your brain first. To nourish the brain, you have to tonify the jing first; to nourish the jing, you have to nourish the blood; to nourish the blood, you will have to nourish the saliva. To achieve all this, you need to nourish your water—the body fluid. The Water Pond is found under the tongue at the point between the two middle teeth. When the Water moves into the lung-channel, it turns into saliva; when it goes into the heart-channel, it turns into blood. The blood then moves into the kidneys, and it will take 250 days to turn into the jing. The jing moves into the brain-channel, forming the Ni Wan Palace (the upper dan tian). In the Ni Wan Palace, there are two channels that move down along the spine and into the Qi hai area (the lower dan tian). When the Qi hai is in charge, the person is lightened up."

Qi energy links all living things to the universe. I have translated the following partial poem written by a female immortal, Celestial Tsao, who defined qi 1,500 years ago in her poem.

> Let me tell you the secret of life,
> The base of life is the zhen (internal) breathing of qi.
> When this starts inside the body,
> Be cautious not to lose it.
> Only when the xin (heart-mind) is carefree, it is your real xin,
> Meditate until forgetting, no matter moving or still,
>   away from anxiety.
> The shen is your nature and the qi is your life source,
> With paying no attention to the outside world, the shen will
>   not be consumed,
> And qi will be calm.
> Shen and qi are originally inseparable,
> To lose them, how can your hold your own root?
> If the primary qi is disturbed,
> Then the shen will not be peaceful,
> And this will be like a worm-eaten tree with no root;
> Its branches and leaves will become withered.
> Talking about snivel, phlegm, saliva, jing, and blood,
> Trace all of these to their source,
> They come from the same thing (fountain).
> This "thing" has no fixed place,
> And it changes according to the mind.
> When your body is hot, it becomes sweat,
> When you are sad, it changes into tears.
> When it works in your kidneys, it changes into the jing,
> But when it goes to your nose, it turns snivel.
> It moves vertically and horizontally
> To moisten the whole body.
> As to what is happening,
> The shen-water will be eventually drained.
> It is difficult to describe this shen-water,
> And people rarely know about it,
> Its production is dependent upon the primary qi,
> Which comes only when you become not indulging in fame,
>   gaining and reduce worries,
> And become a vegetarian with a calm xin and less talking.
> Then one day you will enjoy drinking the "sweet-dew juice,"

And will no longer be hungry and thirsty
As you have discovered the truth of life....
To practice and cultivate relies on the shen and qi,
If the shen and qi are incomplete,
Hard work will be fruitless.
What a pity to this wonderful site of base*
Where a precious house* built of gold and jade yet has no owner.

*The site and house: the body form in metaphor

HOW QI FLOWS IN OUR BODIES

Before you start to practice qigong it is important to get an idea of how qi flows in the body. As you can see in the drawing (Figure 2), qi flows in channels around our bodies. This flow or movement of qi is frequently replenished or diminished by activities such as eating, breathing, expression of emotions, and sleeping. It is even affected by the changes in different hours and seasons. For example, worries, vexations, anxieties, fears, anger, and even extreme joy will affect qi and cause it to flow differently. Located along the qi channels are acupoints. Acupoints are like tiny qi pools that form along the qi channels. These acupoints are often treated by putting needles into them (acupuncture), using moxa (an aromatic medicinal herb) to heat this point or by pressing and massaging this area (acupressure). Each of these methods is used to remove stagnant qi and to adjust the flow of qi.

As the qi flows around our bodies it follows paths such as the Small Heavenly Circle as shown. This path starts at the base of the trunk midway between the vagina and anus, called *Hui yin* point or perineum, and continues up to the back of the body and follows the spine to the top of the head. The path continues from this point down to the forehead, past the roof of the mouth, to the front of the body between the breasts, ending again at the Hui yin. Small Heavenly Circle is one of the main channels. Qi can permeate to all parts of your body by following smaller channels as well. If the large and small channels remain totally unblocked, then the body can be healthy and the practitioner can enjoy a long, healthy life.

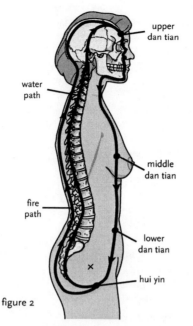

upper
dan tian

water
path

middle
dan tian

fire
path

lower
dan tian

×

hui yin

figure 2

WHAT IS QIGONG AND QIGONG PRACTICE?

As you can see, when you add qi to another Chinese word, *gong,* it forms the word, *qigong.* The word, *qi,* means the life force, and the word, gong, means the experiences and practice that have been handed down. Qigong, therefore, can be translated as "hard work" or "study to learn to induce self-energy, to transfer the energy into usage, or to heal a disease." Qigong is a way to induce energy (qi) that in turn will promote self-healing and long life similar to the way we use electricity to illuminate a light bulb. There are many different styles of qigong and all types include different levels of forms. Elementary levels of any style are mainly used for healing oneself and staying healthy. As you practice and add cultivation, your qi will build up in your body, and sickness will be dispelled. Physical conditions will be improved and emotional states balanced. With more advanced practice, you can increase your ability by mastering and absorbing qi from nature and balancing your mind/heart. Qigong encompasses a great number of things both tangible and intangible, explainable and not.

In short, if we tie all of the above information together, my definition of qigong is fourfold.

1. First and foremost, qigong is the best natural self-healing and life-prolonging science found in the world today. No other such self-preserving health practice has developed into such an integrated, comprehensive effort, merging body, mind, and spirit with physical exercise, medicine, and dietary practices for the preservation of the body and mind.

2. Qigong practice is a self-effort designed to balance and align oneself with nature. It is simple to learn and yet effective in the preservation of physical and emotional health. The practice is a study of the relatedness between human beings, the natural world, and the universe. Because of the nature of qigong, continued practice results in physical and emotional freedoms that allow practitioners to adapt to the world in which we live—in a natural way—much the way qigong helped me to maintain balance and health during my difficult times in my life.

3. Qigong theory is also a cosmic theory. Qigong theory states that because human beings, like all living things on our planet, were produced from qi in the universe, so each part of the human body is then related to the movements of the universe. A familiar yet ancient Taoist symbol, the diagram of the yin and yang, vividly shows the interactions and movements of qi in the universe.

4. Qigong is a science that is too advanced for human beings to completely understand. This should cause scientists and researchers to give it imminent attention.

Qigong practice, proper diet, and medicine are inseparable in their role in preserving health and healing from within. For this reason, all three need cultivation in order to enhance all their efforts in focusing on building up the defense inside your body. Because we live in a highly competitive society, qigong is needed now more than ever. According to traditional Chinese medicine, diseases such as heart disease, cancer, diabetes, and chronic lung problems are caused by mental stress. Emotions such as stress disturb the qi channels and build blockages that plant the seeds of illness. Qigong practice can help; the qi doctor within you will know where to go.

Qigong and Taiji

Qigong practice is an exercise that helps practitioners to become aware of their bodies' internal energy or qi. Because qigong practice sometimes involves slow movements, I am often asked "What is the difference between qigong and taiji?" My answer is, "They are the same. Qigong is the general term for practices that involve the study and cultivation of your body's internal energy; taiji is one type of such practice. However, qigong practice was described much earlier in history. For example, archeological discoveries in the Ma Wang Dui Tomb (206 B.C.-A.D. 220) and a painting on a clay jar found in west China (that archaeologists claimed to be at least 7,000 years old) indicate that qigong was present at those times. Although qigong was first used for health purposes, through the centuries it was integrated into the development of different styles of martial arts and qigong. It is considered the ancestor of the martial arts, both internal and external (e.g., *taiji, gong fu,* and *wushu*). The term, taiji, also comes from the *I Ching.*

Taiji practice is a complete set of forms that includes both aspects of martial arts as well as healing properties. The Immortal Zhang San-feng (A.D. 1368–1644) first publicly taught this practice. Through the centuries, taiji practice developed into three, then five, different styles. Each is named for the family name of the individuals that developed each style. Taiji was introduced to the west a long time before the formal introduction of qigong happened here, so taiji is a more familiar practice in the west.

Types of Qigong

Qigong now often gets classified as either Medical Qigong or Physical Exercise Qigong. These two terms were defined by Chinese officials as a means to conveniently manage and avoid fraud within qigong practice in China. The truth is that all types of qigong fit these two categories, and they can produce the same results and can function in the same capacity.

Qigong practice has both moving and quiet or still forms. The still forms include various types of meditation and can be practiced when sitting, standing, or lying down. A moving form is just that: a form that contains movement. A moving form is a good general purpose starting point for beginners for four reasons:

❖ It will keep your body in shape

❖ The movements are designed scientifically to work on the qi channels inside your body

❖ It will keep your mind free of intrusive thoughts

❖ It will provide exercise for the body and mind that prepares practitioners for learning more advanced qigong techniques.

Both meditation and moving types of qigong work on the internal system, meaning that they help adjust your body to adapt to your own internal changes and to the constant changes in nature such as the four seasons.

QIGONG BREATHING

During qigong practice, natural breathing will eventually turn into deep breathing; this is normal. When breathing deeply try to inhale and exhale deeply and softly, unless it is otherwise specified. Breathing in this way offers more health benefits than the deep breathing from physical exercise. The qigong way of breathing sends qi to the core of your body where life started—the lower dan tian—and to all the channels. After you practice and study for a time, you will see that breathing the qigong way is not simply breathing deeply. Qigong breathing protects your primary qi and absorbs more qi from nature. Eventually, it can become internal breathing like the fetus that breathes inside the mother's womb.

QIGONG EFFECTS

After you practice for a while, you may experience many of the following.

❖ A better appetite with no resulting weight gain. After a long time, you may actually eat less and still retain your normal weight. This is the experience of many qigong practitioners, including myself.

❖ More energy.

❖ Improved health. Qigong practice has special breathing techniques that affect the different organs. (I will explain this in more detail in Chapter 5.)

❖ Slowing down of the aging process. Qigong helps reverse our biological clock. Many qigong practitioners look younger than before they started to practice qigong.

❖ Phenomenal abilities. I have collected much data of such healing and the scientific experiments from the Chinese researchers and hospitals. The potential that qigong practice can bring out of a person remains a phenomenon that modern Western science cannot yet prove. Yet Chinese history demonstrates these phenomena. I have included many examples in my upcoming book, Qigong Phenomena. For example, by practicing qigong, high-level practitioners have preserved their own dead bodies for later generations without them being processed. Some of these natural mummies have been preserved in the temples like the Jiu Hua Mountain Monastery.

Chinese qigong masters and researchers in the hospitals have proved that qigong works whether you believe in it or not. However, if a qigong practitioner believes that practicing will heal, it will speed up the healing process because she has given the freedom to the healer within—her own qi doctor—rather than creating obstacles in her mind that may slow the process.

Qigong and Female Energy

The ancient sages always considered the biological differences between men and women important, and, thus, they made some parts of the practices different for each sex. For example, when laying the palms at lower dan tian, a woman's left palm is placed on top of her right palm, while a man's hands will do the opposite. (The hands specific direction will be described in Chapter 5.)

Immortal Qing Ling (206 B.C.) emphasized that it was more important for a woman to "keep her mind at the heart and to nourish her shen at the *Shan zhong* point" (the point inside, between the two nipples). This point relates to the kidneys and the heart. If a woman keeps her mind at the lower dan tian for a long time, especially when having menses, it will cause heavy menses or leukorrhea (vaginal discharge). Therefore, when you have your menses, your mind should remain empty and relaxed when you practice rather than focused on your lower dan tian.

Because of the differences between the sexes, a Chinese medical doctor will diagnose and treat men and women in very different ways. Examples include:

- ❖ When a Chinese physician examines a man, his qi will be checked first. When checking a female patient, her blood is considered the more important factor.

- ❖ When checking a lung problem, the Chinese medical doctor will feel the female's pulse by focusing on the qi movement in her right lung but will check a male's pulse in the left lung.

- ❖ Even the sex of a fetus can affect the mother's qi to flow differently. If a pregnant woman is ill, the sex of the fetus will determine which herbal remedy the doctor will prescribe. (A traditional Chinese physician can tell the sex of the baby by feeling the mother's pulse. I personally have witnessed this several times.)

Women's biological differences start from day one, even before the sex is distinguished. For example, the *Nanjing Classic* states:

> When the jing (essence) of yin and yang emerges (when the parents' egg and semen emerge), before the fetus changes into different sex, the two kidneys grow first. They are like two halves of a bean, and there is the primary qi in between. The left one is called kidney, the right one is called Ming men (the Life source gate) in which a man's jing is stored, and stores the starting of a woman's egg. When the Ren channel (the front middle channel) grows mature and reaches the xin (heart-mind), the girl's menses comes (at about the age of fourteen). When a boy's Du channel (the middle channel on the back) becomes mature and reaches the kidney, the boy's body begins to produce mature semen (at about the age of sixteen). The primary qi between the kidneys is considered the beginning of life, the origin of the organs, and the root of the twelve main qi channels. Women's bodies begin to age at the age of thirty-five, and men begin to age at forty. If one has kidney deficiency, gray hair grows, and aging starts.

In the Yellow Emperor's *Nei Jing*, it says,

> When treating a difficult illness when the exact area cannot be located, the doctor should use moxa to heat a woman on her Yin qiao, but heat a man on his Yang qiao.

Qiao means point. Yin means female, yang means male. Yin qiao and Yang qiao are two groups of acupoints. The Yin qiao refers to the orificium urethrae. The Yang qiao refers to the ears, eyes, nose and mouth. These points are so named because they go through two different routes, which affect men and women differently.

In China many different experiments have been performed to prove the male/female energy differences. A group of Chinese qigong practitioner-doctor-researchers used one of the oldest Chinese methods to give qi treatment to the feet of a group of men and then to the feet of a group of women. Both groups were examined before and after the treatments. After treatment, the average of the male group's blood circulation was moving slower than that of the female group. Prior to starting the experiment the male group's circulation was moving quicker than the female group. The purpose of doing this experiment was to prove that the ancient Chinese medical practice of treating men and women differently was scientifically based.

Mothers, Babies, and Qigong

Throughout the years I have taught qigong to many American women. I feel it is important that women be informed about qigong practice and children. According to Chinese medical theory, a woman should especially avoid extreme emotions such as anger or sadness when carrying a child because the extreme emotions can harm the child inside her. For example, a sudden shock during pregnancy may cause her child to have epilepsy after the child is born. Excessive grieving can cause qi to be consumed and blockages to form in the Bao channel and blood to appear in her urine. It may cause an abortion or premature childbirth. If the mother is breast feeding, extreme anger or grief can reduce, or even stop, the amount of milk she is producing.

A mother who is a qigong practitioner should learn how to protect her children. Small children practicing moving forms can improve health and intelligence. However, do not encourage a young child to do meditation if there is no qualified teacher nearby. It is easier for a young child to develop some extra sensory (or psychic) powers and your children may, for example, see things that you cannot or develop healing or scanning power. If there is not a good, experienced qigong master to regularly guide and help the child, there can be trouble. The child could lose vitality or become mentally ill. Such incidents have happened to ignorant parents in China.

Immortal Lu Dong-bin (Tang Dynasty, A.D. 618–907) designed a set of forms for women qigong practitioners including forms to help a pregnant women give birth to a gifted child. However, his forms have been handed down only to selected practitioners. (One of the successors was the Immortal Sun, Bu-Er, one of the Seven Immortals mentioned in Chapter 1.)

I hope that this chapter has helped you understand the basic concepts of qigong so that you can better understand what qigong is. The qigong forms you will learn in Chapter 5 are short forms that are especially beneficial to women. It should not surprise you that Chinese researchers and thousands of cancer patients have proven that qigong practice can prevent, regenerate, and heal from inside. Discussions in Chapters 3 through 7 regarding cultivation—working on the heart, diet, Chinese medicine, and qigong—will help you to advance your study and practice of qigong.

Chapter 3

"My life and fate depend on myself, not the Heaven."
—Lao Zi

Cultivation

Cultivation is a process of self-education that can help you gain wisdom by examining your own inner thoughts in order to become a wiser and more self-assured individual. It will help you to become centered, rooted, carefree, peaceful and tranquil. When you begin the cultivation process you will feel the start of such things rapidly, allowing your body to open up so that the healing process can begin. The more you practice cultivation, the more you will protect and nourish your original qi (pre-birth)—the qi from which you were conceived and the qi with which you were born. The most important function of cultivation is that it constantly purifies your qi.

Cultivation is about daily life, and it involves all aspects of your life, such as lifestyle, housing, education, and hobbies like the arts of calligraphy, painting, horticulture, etc. I know this sounds like a whole lifestyle overhaul, but it is not. You can make it simple or complex according to your own situation. For example, I cultivate mainly to examine my inner thoughts and actions, eating habits, and knowledge of herbal medicine. Cultivation is a gradual and growing process that will help you to become more acquainted with yourself. You will see that I have set up this book in a way so that you may incorporate qigong exercises, herbal recipes, and even words of wisdom into your life without causing too much disruption. I know through experience that once you feel the difference it can make in your life, you will further understand how cultivation becomes a life long process. You can incorporate cultivation into your life when making friends, balancing emotions, keeping promises, and understanding the nature of things—even for sexual activity. Cultivation can teach you how to work from the heart to deal with reality and to compromise rather than meet adversity head-on. You will learn to maintain balanced emotions by exercising your emotional heart and exploring your real being to allow you to harmonize with yourself, society, and the natural world.

It is important to note that for the qi to move more vigorously, it needs the body to be totally relaxed so that the channels through which it flows can open up and accept its movement. If you are not relaxed both physically and mentally when practicing qigong, your mind can become confused and disrupt the movement of qi, causing it to send mixed messages to your body. This can cause tension, which in turn can further restrict the movement of qi. Such tension can also cause the body to produce substances that are toxic, and these toxins can then affect your organs and bring about a greater state of imbalance. Consequently, a cycle of harmful events occurs. In our bodies, imbalance can disturb our qi channels and produce the seeds of illness. Eventually these bad seeds if not found early will grow into a "plant," and the symptoms of illness will be displayed. Once planted, the seeds themselves take root in our system long before the "plants" (symptoms) are even seen. Much work will have to be done to eliminate these roots. Throughout the ages, the masters of cultivation have been able to detect these harmful seeds and prevent them from growing. This is why so many believe that health and longevity are related to relaxation and the emotional balancing practice in the Chinese culture. For example, it is believed that prolonged sadness can weaken a person's qi, and that tears of sadness are toxic and should not be swallowed. During a funeral, Chinese men and women are encouraged to cry, but there is a host present whose job is to make sure that crying persons will not "over-grieve" themselves.

Anger and worry are other examples. Excessive anger can harm the liver, which in turn negatively affects the health and functions of the heart. (See Figure 3) When the wood is weak, it cannot produce strong fire. Similarly, if you are worried constantly, you can get a migraine because your disturbed mind has interrupted qi from reaching the nervous system in the head.

You can see why it then becomes important for you to sort out the reason for being mad or upset and to deal with the emotion rather than letting the emotion affect the organ.

Learn to let your inner being be in control, and do not let the mind become polluted. If your mind releases the toxins that pro-

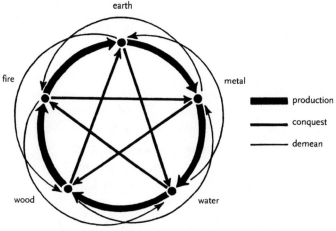

earth

fire

metal

wood

water

production
conquest
demean

figure 3

duced such as stress, then relaxation can allow the healing to continue. Since qigong practice will induce the power of the movement of qi and promote the blood circulation, it is important that
you keep yourself in as relaxed a state as possible when you practice qigong. With the qi moving more vigorously, it needs the body
to be totally relaxed to open up for its movements. When an
extreme emotion is present, however, the mind will increase the
disturbance in the normal circulation of qi. A relaxed state is
essential in assisting your qi cultivation and blood circulation. It
will help you become wiser and deal with emotional disturbances
in a better way. By relaxing, you reverse the cycle, resulting in less
qi blockages and fewer health problems. In truth, the seeds you
subconsciously plant through qigong practice and cultivation can
root out and grow into strong and healthy mind, body, and spirit.

AWARENESS

You can be angry or upset, but if you are aware of it and do
not let such feelings hurt your health, then you are cultivating
your positive feelings. In the words of Confucius, cultivation can
mean, "To examine my inner thoughts and doings three times a
day." In other words, you must be able to be aware of your inner
thoughts—both good and bad—analyze them, and put them into
perspective. This self-check can serve as a means to keep your
thoughts pure and to help you to avoid guilt and ill feelings. It will
also help you keep your mind and heart at peace. When your
mind and heart are at ease, the qi can then be in harmony with
your mind and body. If you have difficulty facing and dealing with

your inner thoughts, you may have difficulty when practicing qigong. It may be more difficult to work on a spiritual level as well. Examination of our thoughts allows us to get to know ourselves better. As you spend time evaluating your thoughts you can gain further insight into the necessity of such thoughts. This process can help you to discover how much time and energy you put into unnecessary thoughts and how that energy is better spent elsewhere. The ancient sage, Lao Zi wrote in the *Tao Te Ching*, "I have three treasures. I cherish them and keep them with me all the time. They are kindheartedness, being thrifty and simple, and not competing with anyone." What he meant is:

❖ Do things in accordance with, and not against, nature.

❖ Hold the shen (spirit) inside so that your vitality will not be wasted.

By practicing qigong and cultivation, I have become aware of my body myself, my thoughts, and how I affect the people with whom I come into contact with each day. I understand that before my body leaves this dimension it needs to become completely physically healthy and run its course. Like all things on our planet, my body needs to love and to be loved (not excessively), to eat to stop hunger, to get nutrition for health, to exercise to stay in shape, to have peaceful thoughts, to live without anxiety. I know that in order to be healthy so that I can explore my inner being, I also need to cultivate, exercise my heart to be more tolerant, and persistently practice qigong. As you have seen by my story, my cultivation has helped me through tough personal and political times in my life. It has been my guide through two marriages, raising children, and dealing with society. Whether I have been sad, happy, or angry, I know that with the inner strength and awareness that I have cultivated through a qigong lifestyle, I have gained the ability to always get my feelings balanced quickly and look to the future. As you become more aware of your cultivation you will understand more of the spirit of qigong, which is just in like a Chinese ancient idiom, "Mud cannot stain lotus, but only nourish its beauty and purity."

Qigong theory is based on compromise, tolerance, and harmony with both the real and the natural world. This spirit will lead you to emotional balance, peace, tranquility, and happiness. The best way to understand the true spirit of qigong is to educate yourself, believe in yourself, and allow yourself to use your own wisdom to make decisions. The qigong spirit penetrates people's lives. In China, there are many people who can tell you how qigong practices have changed them spiritually as well as physically. Qigong practice has even helped some inmates in Chinese prisons to turn over a new leaf when they want to change. Since ancient times there have been stories telling how this spirit has helped people. During turbulent times in Chinese history, officials used the qigong spirit—Taoism—to help establish a more peaceful country. Yin Yi (about 4,000 years ago) carried out the Yellow Emperor's philosophy; his story is included in Chapter 7. Jiang Taigong (about 3,500 years ago) helped the Emperor establish the Zhou Dynasty that lasted 800 years. It was believed that he was one of Lao Zi's reincarnations according to Taoist religion. Zhang Liang (about 2,100 years ago), who helped established the Han Dynasty, was taught by a Taoist Immortal and studied the "Yellow Emperor's Yin Fu Jing." Taoist Kong Ming (about 1,900 years ago, the Three Kingdoms period) helped establish the Han Kingdom.

During the time of Confucius, the King of the Chu Kingdom had difficulty during his reign. He consulted a Taoist grand master, Xin Yi, who was a student of Lao Zi. Xin Yi's advice not only brought the Chu Kingdom out of chaos and the people peace but the kingdom became prosperous and lasted for many years.

The second emperor of the Han Dynasty (206 B.C.–A.D. 220), Emperor Han Wen was raised by a mother who practiced Taoism, so he practiced qigong and Taoism. He ruled China for 24 years, and during his reign he was able to make peace with his political enemies and foreign neighbors without fighting. Almost all the prisons were empty and people lived peaceful lives. The description of the society of his time was written, "No one picked up and pocketed anything lost on the road, and people did not even need to lock their doors." During this time the Silk Road was opened up as well as tea was introduced to the West. China has endured a long, rich, colorful past and in some way the qigong spirit has been present through it all. If you look, you will see many more such examples of how the qigong spirit has touched and changed lives.

CULTIVATION OF QI FOR WOMEN

Up to this point we have been talking about qigong practice and cultivation. Let me first give you a clearer picture of what cultivation of qi is. Cultivation of qi refers to an integration of the whole. It refers not only to the practice of qigong but to becoming more aware of how well you know yourself as an individual, what you think, what you feel, and how you interact with family members, society, as well as what you eat. This self-awareness is important because it all relates to our emotions.

As we already know men and women are different, but these differences go much deeper than the obvious physical ones. For example, according to Chinese medical theory, biologically, men can bathe and shower in cold water, but a woman cannot if she has menses or is pregnant. A man can lift a heavy object, but a woman who has menses or is pregnant cannot. A Chinese physician and qigong master, Jiao Guo-rei, conducted research that says about 70% of illnesses are psychologically related and more of these patients are female that male. These results match the theory found in Chinese traditional medicine that states that many gynecological diseases are related to the emotions. Women also suffer abnormal leukorrhoea, sterility, spasm of the uterus, sexual hyperethesia, bladder problems, tumors and ulcers of uterus, abnormal appetites and menses to name a few, that may be emotionally rooted. I have read studies that state one out of every six of American women suffer migraines that are mainly caused by stress. When you cultivate qi, you can help prevent such illnesses. In order to help you understand this cycle of how things affect each other, I will explain an important theory used in Chinese medicine, diet, and qigong practice: the Five Element Theory. (please refer to Figure 3, p.39)

The five elements are wood, fire, earth, metal and water. The theory is that wood creates fire, fire creates earth, earth creates metal, metal creates water and water creates wood. Ancient Taoist sages used the idea of how the elements interact to explain how qi works in our body, how our organs are related to one another, and how our bodies relate to nature. The interactions of the five elements express a theory of the mutual promotion and restraint between one another, the organs, and how they affect each other.

Additionally, the five elements (Figure 4) provide the guiding principles for many types of qigong practice and for Chinese Medicine and dietary practices. For example, the organs in the body are first classified as either yin (solid) organs and yang (hollow) organs. Each organ is then identified with a particular element (fire, wood, etc.) The organs are not the only things that are associated with the five elements. Taoism and Chinese medicine also associate flavors, colors, seasons, directions, sounds, stars, planets and even our five senses with the five elements as well. Chinese physicians and qigong practitioners have used the application of the Five Element Theory for thousands of years in the prevention of illness and the promotion of longevity.

Ideally, maintaining this balance among the organs in your body will prevent ailments and promote good health and longevity. Understanding this theory becomes important in qigong practice in that its knowledge can aid practitioners to maintain balance within their bodies. For example, when you are angry, the anger can produce toxins in your liver. If you were familiar with the five-element theory, you would know that your liver is associated with the wood element. Additionally, according to this theory water nourishes wood, and your kidneys are associated with the element water. Knowing this, you can then use you qigong practice to detoxify the toxin in your liver first and then send qi to your kidneys, which in turn will nourish your liver and remove the anger, and thus, put your body and mind back in balance.

	WOOD 木	FIRE 火	EARTH 土	METAL 金	WATER 水
DIRECTION	East	South	Center	West	North
SEASON	Spring	Summer	Long Summer	Autumn	Winter
CLIMACTIC CONDITION	Wind	Summer Heat	Dampness	Dryness	Cold
PROCESS	Birth	Growth	Transformation	Harvest	Storage
COLOR	Green	Red	Yellow	White	Black
TASTE	Sour	Bitter	Sweet	Pungent	Salty
SMELL	Goatish	Burning	Fragrant	Rank	Rotten
YIN ORGAN	Liver	Heart	Spleen	Lungs	Kidneys
YANG ORGAN	Gall Bladder	Small Intestine	Stomach	Large Intestine	Bladder
OPENING	Eyes	Tongue	Mouth	Nose	Ears
TISSUE	Sinews	Blood Vessels	Flesh	Skin/Hair	Bones
EMOTION	Anger	Happiness	Pensiveness	Sadness	Fear
HUMAN SOUND	Shout	Laughter	Song	Weeping	Groan

Figure 4

Some may laugh but the phrase "Do not worry, be happy" is good medicine for good health in any culture. According to qigong theory, a peaceful mood will produce yang qi that is beneficial to your health. There is a Chinese saying "Laughter can reduce ten years of aging." Even when Chinese people try to stop two people from fighting, they would say, "You two please have an even-tempered and good-humored talk." (The spoken language is: *Xin ping qi heh*: "easing-minded and qi-harmonized") I have translated a poem to show you an example of how to retain a peaceful mind. Perhaps when you are dealing with things that upset you, the words in this poem may help you deal with them better. This poem was written by a high official who was a qigong practitioner. He lived a healthy life for one hundred years.

"Song of Avoiding Getting Angry"
—*Yuan Jing-ming*

When another person gets angry, but not me,
Because I did not wish to cause his anger.
If I was upset as he was,
Only an illness would be caused in me.
It is difficult for a doctor to treat a patient who holds anger,
So being not angry is what I am always cautious to be.
Anger can cause a person ill, and even could cause his or her life,
This is what I have learned from life,
No matter what I am not angry,
No anger and will not get angry.

EATING TO CULTIVATE QI

As I started to write this book, I knew immediately that I did not want to write a book of only qigong exercises. Rather I wanted to write a book that would give you an idea how to make positive changes in your life through qigong practice and cultivation. Eating is an important factor in cultivation. "Qi is the commander of blood" is a Chinese medical theory meaning qi leads the blood circulation. If the qi movement is disturbed it will affect the blood circulation and then health problems may result. The self-education of eating right will teach you to eat in harmony with qi, so as not to disturb the qi circulation inside our bodies. Therefore, not eating right can disturb your qi and then affect your emotions and health. I have seen so many people harming themselves unknowingly in this country simply because they are not aware of what they are putting into their bodies. So many people eat unhealthy fast foods on the run day after day. First of all they are not taking the time to digest properly, and, secondly, they are eating the same processed foods day after day. To the Chinese, balance is always emphasized in diet. They are aware of what and when they are eating and are mindful to give sufficient time to allow the body to digest the food. Most Chinese people do not allow themselves to become addicted to a certain flavor or type of food, because different flavors affect different organs. For example, sourness affects the liver, bitterness affects the heart, sweetness affects the spleen, etc. Additionally, different types of food benefit different organs. In short, if one becomes addicted to one kind of flavor or one type of food, this excessiveness can become harmful to one of the organs and neglect the others, thus causing a chain-reaction effect within your body. When one organ loses balance, the shen (spirit) will be disturbed. If this happens, the shen will not be able to guide the qi to circulate it in the normal way.

Not only does food affect our bodies, but also the effects of foods will vary from person to person because age, gender, and health condition differ between individuals. Thus, it becomes important that you know your own body so that you can recognize if something is wrong.

It is very important for you to educate yourself in the area of eating so that you can eat in harmony with both your body's own makeup and your surroundings (such as the seasons and even geographic location). Doing so will help prevent illness, heal sickness, and keep you healthy. According to Chinese medicine, foods all have different natures that affect our bodies in different ways. One needs to acquire a basic knowledge about the different natures and functions of various foods and herbs, such as the difference between dark and white sugar or between the calcium made from animal bones or oysters. In the hot summer, for example one will learn that to release the summer heat from inside is more important than cooling down in air conditioning. By drinking some boiled mung bean tea, hot green tea, or lotus seed-heart tea—or eating watermelon— you can release internal heat allowing your body to cool from the inside out. If people knew that drinking any one of the above drinks would work on the qi inside the body to prevent and soothe some hidden causes of heat (air conditioning does not address these causes), illness and deaths caused by excessive heat would be reduced. Practicing this kind of scientific eating is vital to the flow of qi and is, considered part of cultivation. Working on the qi inside the body can prevent and heal some of the hidden causes of distress and disease that, once the external symptom has surfaced, may be too advanced to treat properly.

I will discuss such ways of eating in Chapter 7, but do not rely solely on me for such information. Take the initiative in your own education process. If you have Internet access, browse the web for sites concerning healthy eating or the use of herbs in food preparation. Check you local library for books or magazines concerning well-balanced eating, eating meals for preserving health, and diet for healing different diseases. With your own wisdom and education, you will be able to choose helpful, correct information. There are a large quantity books of food recipes for health and longevity purposes in China, and some have been translated into English. Try to find such books and add to you self-education process. Books concerning herbology or herb lore and traditional Chinese medicine may help you better understand the benefits of eating correctly.

EMOTIONAL BALANCE

We live in a highly competitive society. In such a society we can suffer from mental stress that can cause many diseases, such as heart disease, cancer, diabetes, and chronic lung problems, to name a few. Each day we can face emotional disturbances that are difficult to handle or that are disturbing to us. Cultivation can help you cope with situations so they become less difficult to handle. Through cultivation you can learn not only how to cleanse your body of toxins produced by extreme emotions, but also to lessen or eliminate the amount you produce. Such a process can help you balance your mind, body, and spirit by teaching you to turn to yourself and your own internal energies rather than letting your emotions get the best of you.

Please do not misunderstand me. Expressing and experiencing emotion is natural and not necessarily detrimental to your well-being as long as it is not done in excess. If you listen to ancient Chinese music or look at the paintings of the ancient times you will notice that they are quite soothing to the ears and eyes. Even the subject matter of ancient Chinese poetry is that of nature and the reader's relationship to it. All of this was done to promote a calm and tranquil setting. The idea of keeping emotional balance is best exemplified in the yin and yang diagram. (please refer to Figure 1, p.22, Yin and Yang diagram)

If you look closely at the yin and yang diagram, you will see that when yang (white) is at its most extreme or widest point the yin (black) begins or is at its thinnest. Thus, extreme yang gives rise to the beginning of yin and vice versa. According to yin/yang theory, this is the state of all things. If we apply this theory to emotions and health, we can conclude that extreme emotions can cause poor health, and poor health can make a person extremely emotional and the cycle will continue repeating itself, perhaps resulting in premature death. A Chinese idiom states, "When shen is calm, qi becomes clear." Therefore, it becomes important that you also realize the importance of retaining a balanced emotional state, which is what qigong practice and cultivation can help you to attain. Purity is an important state of your heart that only comes from cultivation, which is the most important stage in more advanced qigong practice.

I would like to conclude this chapter with the advice of a father to his children, and also my translation from a well-known Taoist, *Gao Lian*. The father's name is Li Hong-zhang who was the Prime Minister who served several weak emperors and a very difficult Empress. In spite of difficulties Li achieved some success and lived for eighty years because he practiced qigong and cultivation.

> *The illness can only happen to the physical body, but not to the will of xin (mind/heart). If a person's body is ill, his will of xin should not be ill. Then what the sickness can do to him? If one has fame, wealth, and also is an outstanding scholar, but he is not in good health, then none of them will be useful. That is why one must know how to preserve health.*

TRANSLATIONS

One Hundred Illnesses

—*Gao Lian*

("*Water*" *and* "*fire*" *in the poem represent the kidneys and heart. Losing balance between them results in dysphoria, insomnia, and nocturnal emission.*)

To be overjoyed or excessively angry is an illness,

To take without justice is an illness,

To indulge in sex without morality is an illness,

To be obsessed loving one person is unhealthy,

To dislike sex with no reason is an illness,

To give way to the carnal desires, greediness, and cover up one's own wrongdoings is a sickness,

To attack others in order to build up oneself is a sickness,

To be very shrewd for inventing excuses for oneself is an illness,

To talk a lot and give promises easily is an illness,

To follow wrongdoings for pleasure is a sickness,

To look down upon others by relying on resourcefulness is a sickness,

To abuse power and behave recklessly is a sickness,

To think of oneself never being wrong is an illness,

To bully widows, young children, and weak and helpless people is an illness,

To win by force is a sickness,

To intimidate people with power or influence is an illness,

To always win in a conversation is an illness,

To borrow money but not want to pay it back is an illness,

To wrong others so as to vindicate oneself is not healthy,

To speak honestly yet hurting others is a sickness,

To make friends with evil people is an illness,

To harm oneself by being overjoyed or angry is unhealthy,

To think of self as extraordinary although not a smart person is unhealthy,

To be arrogant and imperious because of merits and achievement is not healthy,

To slander well-known people who have good virtue is a sickness,

To complain and blame self because of overworking is not healthy,

To believe in lies as the truth is an illness,

To enjoy finding faults of others and criticize is a sickness,

To despise others because of being rich is an illness,

To ridicule the noble people because of having a low social status is a sickness,

To frame someone else in order to ingratiate with a person in power is a sickness,

To show off because of being morally good is an illness,

To look down upon others because of holding high position is an illness,

To be jealous of the rich because being poor is an illness,

To ruin someone's success is a sickness,

To use others as ladders for self-achievement is a sickness,

To use authority for private benefits is a sickness,

To like to cover up one's own wrongdoings and mistakes is an illness,

To put others in danger for one's own safety is an illness,

To be jealous and unreliable is a sickness,

To hold extreme views and be aggressive and angry is an illness,

To hate more and love less and the love is limited is unhealthy,

To go on arguing for the sake of arguing and fight physically is an
   illness,
To shift blame on others is a sickness,
To speak sweet words for private gains is a sickness,
To gossip behind others' back is an illness,
To fool people under false pretenses using powerful names is an illness,
To help someone and expect to be paid back is unhealthy,
To blame others without helping is a sickness,
To regret after giving is unhealthy,
To secretly complain and hate is a sickness,
To enjoy killing animals, bugs, and worms is a sickness,
To confuse and poison others' minds by witchcraft is a sickness,
To calumniate talented and outstanding people is an illness,
To hate others when they are better than self is a sickness,
To enjoy taking toxic things and poisonous drink is a sickness,
To think of people unequally is an illness,
To delude the kindhearted, worthy people with fallacies and rumors is a
   sickness,
To cherish the memory of the bad things that one did is an illness,
To refuse advice and criticism of one's faults is a sickness,
To be close with others but distant from family members is a sickness,
To write letters to discredit others is an illness,
To laugh at disabled people is a sickness,
To be easily fidgety, harsh, rash, and restless is an illness,
To often hit fists on the table angrily and unreasonably is an illness,
To love being in control and the boss is unhealthy,
To be very suspicious and have no trustworthiness is a sickness,
To laugh at mentally ill people is a sickness,
To be rude and impolite to people is a sickness,
To talk in dirty and vicious language is a sickness,
To treat old people and children without proper respect is a sickness,
To argue rudely and use vicious abusive language is an illness,
To be self-willed, ruthless and tyrannical is a sickness,
To love to laugh loudly and be excessive in joy is a sickness,
To be in power and let oneself go is an illness,
To be treacherous, fawn on, and ingratiate is a sickness,
To indulge in gaining with a cheating and cunning mind is a sickness,
To be a double-dealer, go back on one's word, and not be trustworthy is
   a sickness,
To play the tyrant taking advantage of being drunk is unhealthy,
To swear at the weather changes is a sickness,
To enjoy speaking abusively and killing people is an illness,
To teach others abortion is a sickness,
To intervene into others' personal business is a sickness,

To make a hole to peek into other people's life is an illness,

*To harbor resentment because of being refused when borrowing is a
sickness,*

To run away from debts is a sickness,

To talk differently behind other people's backs is unhealthy,

*To like arguing with fierce, brutal, arrogant, rude, and unreasonable
people is unhealthy,*

To assail women with obscenities is a sickness,

*To purposely cause delay and hurt to others by pretending to make
mistakes is a sickness,*

To damage the bird's net when searching for eggs is an illness,

*To be in big shock and then harm the fetus and cause an abnormal
birth is an illness,*

*To breakdown the balance between the water [kidneys] and fire [heart]
to harm one's own health is unhealthy,*

To make fun of blind, mute people is a sickness,

To interfere in others' marriage is a sickness,

To incite violence is a sickness,

To teach others to do evil things is an illness,

*To run away from loved ones because of stirring up trouble is a
sickness,*

To praise disaster and wrongdoings is an illness,

To be out for small advantages is unhealthy,

To forcibly seize others' belongings is a sickness.

Above are one hundred kinds of illnesses. If you can get rid of all
of them, and examine your thoughts and behaviors, there will be no
disaster, pain, worries, dangers, and critical conditions. You will not
only preserve good health and longevity, but also protect your later
generations by the happiness that you have created for them.

In addition to the above, making friends with good people is
also important to cultivation because their qi energy field is positive and they are a good emotional influence. The ancient sages
(and some qigong masters today) were able to see the different
colors of qi in different people. The good-hearted people give off
sky blue qi. The following translation comes from ancient China
and is concerned with the importance of making friends.

High from the emperors, down to the ordinary people, no one can be successful without friends. However, in this society, there are also some fraudulent people and villains. How can I tell first that he is a good person or not? My ways is, if he is crafty and spies on me, I am decent and honest and he cannot find what he is looking for. If he is greedy and wants me to fail, he will not get anything because I will not fail. He cannot get me interested in the things that I like to do for his own purpose. If we are in a conversation, I only talk about the right things with him. I will not listen to the words that he tries to slander me, and they will not influence my mind. If I can supply a good meal and eat with him, I will not be lured by his suggestions to mess up my own business. If I am unselfish, how can he influence me with seeking private gains? I am well on guard and armed with my own weapons, what man-made trouble can harm me?

A friend who has only a friendly face but not from the heart is called "facial friend" (false friend).

A friend who is not greedy but courageous and does not believe in gossip will be a life-long friend.

When friends are together, they straighten each other, when apart,

They talk nice things about each other; when one is enjoying something, he thinks of the other; when one is sick, the other will be very sad.

When a friend takes from you, you can trust him not to be greedy; when he runs away, you know that he is not a coward.

As friends, when they hold hands to have a whole-hearted conversation, they encourage family bounding, respect their parents, help to bound the relationship between the husband and wife, the father and son's closeness, and the care between brothers and sisters, etc.

If a person does not cultivate, it is his owns fault; if a person cultivates but still has a bad name, it is his friend's fault. This is why at home, he should cultivate, and going out, he will make friends with nice people.

Also on friends:

A person who has self-knowledge is wise and will not blame other people;

A person who knows his or her fate (where life comes from) does not complain about the Heaven.

—Xun Zi

Chapter 4

One grown in the understanding of Tao (the Way).
            —Master Liu Qing-yuan

How to Start

As you continue your qigong journey it is a good idea to integrate both moving forms and meditation into your practice so that you can make more progress by balancing your mind and body. A well-known Chinese fable written by the sage, Zhuang ze (369–298 B.C.) tells us the tale of two individuals who did not heed this advise.

> One man named Shan Bo practiced only the inner qigong (quiet forms such as sitting meditation). His inner organs were healthy, his skin was fine and he looked very young at the age of seventy, but physically he was not strong. One day, a tiger attacked him. With no strength to fight, the tiger ate him. Another man named Zhang Yi, only practiced muscle-building exercise (only physical exercise, like body-building) and was very strong physically. He sought out fame and money. Possessing no inner strength he became ill at the age of thirty and died soon after.

These fables are great examples of just how long the concept of balance has been integrated into the Chinese society and why it is so important to cultivate it. Building only physical strength and prowess can leave an individual with little mental stimulation. On the other hand, practicing only meditation can leave our bodies weak and feeble. In either case you may suffer. The key is balance. Only with a good sense of balance in your life can you benefit from the best of cultivating both sides.

Learn a formal qigong form from a teacher that has good resources so that the form you are taught has been designed and handed down by great masters. Such a form should possess beginning, intermediate, and advanced levels. Regardless of the type of qigong you are practicing, it is always important to have good resources to guide you on your journey. Do not be afraid to ask questions. If a good teacher is not available in your area, seek out as much information as you can so that you can be clear about what you are doing. Try to attend a seminar or conference so that you may find others with whom you can discuss qigong. You need to be sure that what someone is trying to teach you is, in fact, the real thing and not something that they know a little about or perhaps made up.

No matter how simple a form may appear, discussion and practice with experienced teachers and practitioners can help you to make progress that you may not accomplish on your own. Remember though, the key here is practice. You can discuss these concepts all you want, but you cannot and will not make progress without practice. Without practice you will be like "swimming on land," and you will get nowhere fast. In the spirit of qigong it is up to you and you alone to practice and study to make the changes in your life that you desire. For advanced practice, I suggest you seek a good teacher. The short forms I include in Chapter 5 are for your education and to help specific needs. They are short so that they can fit into your busy schedule so that you can keep you "qi-engine" going.

There is a vast ocean of qigong forms that you can learn, but there is a difference between accumulating forms and mastering them. As a beginner, it is a good idea for you to gather plenty of knowledge, but remember that the key to success here is quality not quantity. By writing this book, I am trying to give you a basic understanding of all that makes up the practice of qigong. However, as you become more familiar with qigong practice you will see the vastness of it. This is where I hope that you remember to cultivate the basics and do them well. Choose a basic form and stick to it; practice persistently so that you have a good solid foundation. Only then will you have an idea if you are making progress. If you try too many things all at once, you will be unable to tell what is working and what is not. Do not mix the movements of different forms because this may cause trouble to your health since each type is designed to approach healing differently. We all have individual differences and preferences so it becomes important to find which type of qigong works for you.

Having a solid foundation in basic qigong practice and theory will be your guide as your practice begins to make progress. In 1998, I met an individual in the United States who was a practitioner of Soaring Crane Standing Meditation. He had stopped practicing because of an incident that happened to him that he did not understand, and he did not choose to seek an answer. He told me that as he was practicing the standing meditation one day he suddenly felt as if he was enveloped in clouds and could see nothing. He became scared and stopped practicing. I told him it was too bad that he stopped practicing because he missed a big step in his qigong journey. If he had the proper guidance during his cultivation he may have understood what was happening to him, and his experience could have empowered him in further practice. Instead, he stopped his practice all together. Please do not misunderstand me. I do not mean to lead you to believe that you will have such experiences. What I do mean is that, as a beginner, you need to obtain a good foundation of knowledge and support so that if you experience subtle changes in your body you will recognize them as such and continue to practice. Do not be afraid to seek wisdom. Read and become as knowledgeable as you can. Do remember, however, that all of the ancient books written by the sages were compiled from their own personal experiences so that their practice became tailored to their own characters; the masters designed various types of qigong in order to accommodate different individuals. Only through knowledge and practice will you gain enough understanding about yourself so that you too can make progress. Practice persistently for the sake of practice, and put aside the desire of results. Doing so will lead you to progress.

I am often asked the question, "Is one time of day better than another to practice?" According to the ancient texts the various times of the day are related to the different organs of the body. However, practicing whenever you have time is beneficial. I personally like to absorb qi in the morning, do the moving during my break time, and meditate late at night. I also try to maintain my qigong state in daily activities. Simply put: choose to practice according to your own lifestyle and pace.

When you are first learning to practice qigong, learn the movements first. Remember to touch the tip of your tongue to the roof of you mouth directly behind your teeth so that you keep the connection closed as the qi flows around your body.

As a beginner, you may encounter common misunderstandings that often occur as you begin your practice. I will try to introduce to some of the more common ones in an effort to provide you with a good starting point. Some common mistakes that can occur in the beginning are:

- The practitioner focuses too attentively on only one point of the body or focuses at only one area for a long time.

- The practitioner becomes creative or mixes the forms when practicing.

- The practitioner experiences a healing sensation like numbness, soreness, pain, or cold sweats—and stops practicing. Do not be concerned; these responses in your body are normal. This is because the qi-doctor is pushing and fixing your body. If you remain relaxed the sensation will disappear.

- The practitioner loses faith or grows impatient and changes forms frequently. You will not make progress this way. Immortal Lu said that such a practitioner was like a snake that had two heads; each head wants to go to his own way and will never get anywhere.

- The practitioner has a strong wish of being cured, making progress, or producing longevity. When this happens, her xin will not be relaxed or clear, but rather like a cup of water with floating sands.

I have met practitioners in the United States that expect a miracle from a qigong master's treatment but at the same time forget their own self-effort in practice. In China, all the patients who received qigong treatments also practice certain types of qigong in order to help themselves. They realize the importance of helping themselves by helping the doctor.

There are no time limitations on how long to practice but you should practice at least one or two times a day. If you practice persistently but desire nothing, you will attain the best results. I can describe it best as growing crops and working hard, but not expecting grains. Then, you will be most successful.

Making self-judgments is important when practicing, as is choosing the right environment, situation, and food. It is also important to understand how to handle the physical changes, including making the right choice among the various qigong books.

Try to pay attention to the wording written in the forms that you are practicing. When you are asked to close your eyes, it means not to just physically close your eyes but to keep out the outside world. Try to keep your mind peaceful and forget the real world. The same holds true for the term "relax." This means relax everything—mind and body, part by part—so that there is no tension within you. When you begin to practice the form, follow the steps as closely as you can. Each movement is there for a reason. As you continue to practice, these reasons will become more apparent.

I have chosen to discuss briefly in this chapter about only a few forms in order to acquaint you with their origin. Much information is readily available via book or Internet to help instruct you in a qigong practice. Much of what I have compiled together in this book is not readily available in one place. I brought it together to help the beginning qigong practitioner integrate qigong into her (or his) lifestyle. The styles that I have chosen to discuss are only the few practices that are promoted by the Qigong Association of America. More widely known qigong long forms also exist and are also reliable. For example, Soaring Crane Qigong and Fragrant (or Aromatic) Qigong have been passed on by grand masters that have many years of experience teaching millions of students in China. These forms are well suited for beginners and are great for promoting healing. According to reports in 1995, Soaring Crane has over 20 million students and Fragrant Qigong has over 90 million practitioners worldwide.

Soaring Crane Qigong began to gain popularity in China when the Cultural Revolution was ending in the 1970s. During that time, many people were ill and sought help. The political atmosphere was loosening up a bit on qigong practice, so Master Zhao Jin-xiang began to teach people in the park. Since then, this qigong practice has helped millions of people and has gained popularity. Master Zhao himself healed his own multiple severe illnesses through the practice of this qigong. I was taught this particular form from Professor Chen, Hui-xian who was one of the dying cancer patients whose life was saved by this qigong. The Soaring Crane Qigong promotes mind balance and provides physical activity for the body. The physical movements associated with this form also help to promote healthy joints such as the neck joints and the shoulders. The movements of this form exercise the acupoints on your back that your hands cannot reach, such as the point, *Gao huang*, that is used to treat all types of illnesses. This form also helps knees (that age quickly) and feet (that carry the weight of your body). The form's advanced version, the Soaring Crane Standing Meditation, is a form not usually taught to beginners because it may be too advanced for a beginner. Frankly, you may need additional guidance. This is why a beginner must seek a good teacher with whom to practice.

In the summer of 1996, I injured my lower back by carrying some heavy object and could not stand more than three minutes at a time. Because I was in pain I had to lie down most of the time. I practiced

Soaring Crane Standing Meditation for less than an hour each day to readjust the joints. Within three days, my back was cured.

Another popular qigong exercise is Fragrant Qigong. According to Tian Rui-shen, the Grand Master of Fragrant Qigong, this practice was handed down by a successor of the Lord Buddha, named Lian Huan Shen who first taught Buddhism in Tibet. Later successors in each generation were either Monks or Taoists, all depending on their qualifications.

Fragrant Qigong works very well especially for seniors and children because the movements are simple and easy to learn and it requires little mind work. Its movements, especially at its second level, also exercise important joints, such as the lower back and knees. When my son was in high school, he would exercise this form whenever he caught a cold. He likes to practice this form when he has a cold because he can watch TV at the same time (in a relaxed state, though). I always felt the sick, cold qi discharge from his fingers when he practiced.

I also taught my in-laws this form during the Christmas season in 1996. During the first month, the pain in my mother-in-law's leg (pain from three surgeries) disappeared, and my father-in-law told me that he "began to sleep like a log." Ever since then, these two seniors have been persistently exercising once a day.

Qigong practice is finally beginning to spread throughout the world, and more and practitioners are reaping the benefits. In France and other European countries, as well as the United States, the set of Jade Body Qigong is gaining popularity. This form was created by Grand Master, Dr. Liu Dong who did the AIDS experiments in collaboration with a well-known French scientist. In Russia and Ukraine, the Zhong Yuan Qigong System has been taught for ten years and is spreading into Europe and the United States. Its Grand Master Xu, Ming-tang, (also known as Misha) has done very impressive qi experiments in collaboration with Ukrainian scientists. Both these two young masters have profound qigong knowledge and have explored their extra sensors. Whatever form you choose to learn, any of the above mentioned formats can help you get started

Chapter 5

Enjoy a free, leisure day
as a fortune.
– Nan Huai-jin

Short Forms

INTRODUCTION

Like traditional Chinese herbal medicine or any other natural healing system qigong does not work in the same way as drugs used in western medicine so one needs to be patient when healing a chronic problem. Remember the natural healing process takes time and is also dependent on the severity of the injury or ailment. Therefore, for most cases, you may not experience a quick fix with this method. Your health will, however, improve over time and you will be on your way to the prevention of further illness. When using qigong as a healing tool, you will become more comfortable and confident with yourself. This will allow you to be more relaxed as you practice so that the healing can continue more readily. I have used qigong with successful results to heal some problems that have arisen in my life.

When my daughter was about three years old, I accidentally hit my left hip hard on a sharp table corner. Years later that spot began to give me an uncomfortable feeling when I sat for too long or when my leg was not warm enough. This injury caused damage to my sciatic nerve. For many years, it was only a discomfort so I just tolerated it and did not give it much thought. I guess, as we all tend to do, I neglected my own problems because something else was more important. Finally, one day after working at the computer all morning I decided to take a break around two in the afternoon to practice meditation. When I started, I was able to relax and let go of my distractions easily that day. As I continued to practice, though, that area of my hip started to ache and gradually the ache increased into pain. At this point, I made the decision to continue my practice because I realized that the healing process was beginning. The pain finally became so bad that I was almost doubled over. I somehow knew that I might be experiencing some sort of breakthrough. Finally the pain became so intense that I almost could not bear it, but I was aware that this was a healing process. I tried to remain in a carefree state and not to pay much attention to the pain. I remembered not to clench my teeth so as not to block my kidney energy (according to Chinese medicine, the kidneys can open and close). By not closing my teeth, the energy would flow. I felt a strong qi force gathering in that area, and then it was trying to push through. While the pain was still intense I felt a whirling sensation where the pain was and then the pain quickly and suddenly was gone. At that moment, my hip felt ever so good and relaxed. Ever since then, the discomfort that I had always had in my hip is gone. The healing process seemed to last a long time, yet in reality it was only a few minutes. Sometimes when I sit at the computer for too long, I experience a gentle warning that it is time to get up and stretch so that I do not get stiff. At this point, I stand up and walk around a little, and then I am all right. The main thing is that I no longer experience the nagging discomfort that I endured for so long. It was through my qigong practice that I was able to overcome my problem, but it did not happen overnight either.

The healing processes and experiences differ from person to person. Some heal gradually over time and some have experiences like mine. Yet, those who do experience the healing qualities of qigong all possess the confidence that they are able to heal themselves.

The practice of qigong can be very flexible so that it can easily fit into your particular lifestyle. Qigong practice will help you to reach a more carefree state and approach your inner being where healing and prevention begins. It will also build your ability to adapt your body to nature's way, which allows for a more natural existence. Qigong should not be practiced merely for healing an injury or illness, although it certainly can be used in such a capacity. Qigong practice and cultivation can open you up to the world of preventive medicine.

As I have mentioned earlier, in the world of qigong practice there is a large variety of forms that can be studied. Included in that multitude are a tremendous number of short forms that can be incorporated into your daily life as well. These short forms are designed to promote balance in your life and many of them are also designed to help along a particular illness or injury that pertains to being uniquely female. In addition to helping an injury or illness, many of these short forms can be practiced during the day to help you continuously maintain a carefree qigong state. This, in turn, will benefit your health and keep your qi "engine" running in the event that it is impossible to take the time to practice a long form. The following forms that I have translated are from Buddhist Grand Master Yuan Huan-xian, Grand Master and Dr. Yan Xin, and the texts of the ancient qigong-master physicians, Tao Hong-jing (A.D. 452–536), Sun Si-miao (A.D. 581–682), and Chao Yuan-fang (A.D. 586–618). I have arranged the forms according to the time of day when they can be practiced for general well-being or according to a particular problem that you might be experiencing. Read through them and feel free to select a form that best suits the needs of your own lifestyle. Each of the following short forms can be practiced as solo forms as well as to compliment a long form.

When you practice any qigong form, it is not good to focus your mind solely on one area of the body or to focus at only one area for a long period of time. It is also more important to feel what you are doing when you are practicing than worrying about the movements.

I have selected three qigong exercises that can be done first thing in the morning depending on how much time you have before starting your daily routine. This qigong should be done after you wake up before you get out of bed.

In the Morning

Roll on your right side. Try to remain in the relaxed state of awakening. Lay your two hands together, left half palm on top of right palm. Place them near your face with fingers pointing to the head of your bed. Touch the tip of your tongue to the roof of your mouth directly behind your teeth. Place your left leg on top of your right and bend the left leg slightly so that the left foot is still touching the lower portion of your right leg. Try to keep your body relaxed. Allow saliva to collect in your mouth and gently swallow it. Try to trace its path in your mind as it goes down your middle qi channel to your lower dan tian. Do not allow yourself to fall asleep. Remain relaxed and keep your mind vaguely at the lower dan tian. When you are ready to get up, knock your teeth together several times to exercise and firm the teeth and to get your body out of the meditating state. Swallow saliva again to follow its path to the lower dan tian to condense qi there. When you have finished, get up slowly and begin your daily tasks.

If you have your menses, simply empty your mind and relax rather than focusing your mind at your lower dan tian.

If you have more time, after completing the above exercise, rather than getting up from bed, roll on to your back stretch your arms above your head and legs downward, thinking all the joints including your spine are pulled apart slightly and relaxed. Focus your mind on taking a long deep breath and inhale. As you exhale say the word, "heh," softly and relax the whole body. Repeat three times. This helps release filthy qi from your chest.

Next roll on your left side in the same way as before, and swallow saliva and trace its path with your mind to the lower dan tian and remain there for a minute. Roll back over on to your back and rub your hands together until hot, place the index and middle fingers on either side of your nose, rub up and down massaging this area for about one minute. Rubbing hot hands in this area helps with the qi circulation because our hands bring qi to the area that you massage. Now, sit up. Using your fingers tap your eyes gently on the eyeballs with your eyes closed for a minute to improve the vision. Then grab your ears between your thumb and forefingers and gently pull them down and up then move them forward and back, for about a minute. Next place your palms over your ears so that they cover your ears tightly and your fingers rest on the back of your head. Place your index finger on top of your middle finger and snap your index finger off your middle finger so that it taps the back of your head. Do this 24 times. This tapping is called, "beating the drum of Heaven" and will help to improve your hearing. After you have completed the drumming section, remain quiet for a minute then quickly massage your face with your palms and fingers in the way that you wash your face. This is another good stopping point if your morning time is limited and you may get up slowly and begin you daily routine.

If you have more time, after completing the above exercise, sit up in bed in a crossed leg meditation posture (if your bed is soft find a more suitable place) for as long as you wish. Be sure to keep your back straight and your head level. Keep your chin slightly tucked so that you have good posture. Circle your tongue first inside and then outside your teeth in a clockwise and counterclockwise manner to massage your gums. When you do this saliva will collect in your mouth swallow small amounts of it three times. When you swallow imagine the saliva as water rinsing your internal organs as it makes its way to the lower dan tian. This helps improve the functions of the organs and prevents aging.

If you still have time, practice either your moving form or the Six Ways of Exhaling (described later in this chapter).

Although this short qigong form is commonly done in the morning, all of the facial massage from this exercise can be done anytime during the day to help relieve stress and tension and is not limited to morning practice.

At Work

In many instances once we leave our homes and enter the workplace all of our comfort feelings that we experience at home go right out the window. For your emotional as well as physical well-being it is important that you make time to bring the relaxation that qigong promotes to the workplace even if it is for a few moments at a time during your busy day.

This short form is good to practice if your job requires a lot of mental concentration and less physical activity. Once you settle in at work but before you start working, take a minute to relax your body and mind. Try this visualization; imagine a candlelight in your heart area for a minute, try to focus your thoughts and energies in this area and focus at the light. Then slowly focus back on your surroundings and begin your work, but keep a little awareness at the light in your chest during the day. When your work is completed turn your focus back to your heart for a minute or two before leaving your workplace. This practice helps keep your shen (spirit) inside so that you will not drain much energy.

If your job does not take your full concentration, try to pay a little more attention to your heart or keep that notion in the back of your mind while you are doing your work. When you take a break inhale and exhale in the qigong way: deeply, softly, and continuously. With each inhalation, gently swallow your saliva and visualize it going to the lower dan tian.

When You are Walking

1. You can try this if you are just walking to get from place to place or if you are out for a daily walk for exercise. As you walk, try to keep your pace comfortable and steady but not fast. Let your thoughts flow from your mind so as to keep out distractions and focus your attention to your heart area. Try to create a rhythm with your breathing as you walk. Inhale through the nose and exhale through the mouth when the air is fresh. You can try to count as you inhale and exhale so as to lengthen your breaths. With each inhalation visualize gently sending qi to the lower dan tian to store more vital energy.

2. If the air is fresh where you are walking visualize all the pores of your body opening up when you inhale slowly and softly. Then hold your breath gently as long as you can, and, at the same time, visualize qi being absorbed into your spine. Before you exhale, you swallow some saliva. Follow it first to the lower dan tian and then visualize all your pores closing. Finally, exhale through your mouth slowly and softly. You may repeat this as many times as you like. As you practice this form, breathing softly, gently, and evenly is important.

3. If you walk in an area where the air is not fresh and clean such as in a hospital, do not practice breathing exercises and you will not inhale much harmful air. As you walk in this type of environment, visualize a fireball in your heart area. This will help protect you body from absorbing external toxins.

4. The following Taoist form is effective for helping you both increase your walking speed and endurance and balance the qi in your body. If you are out on a long hike, walk, or run you can add this qigong practice to your journey to help you to stay alert and invigorated along the way. Visualize the sun shining on your back, the moon shining on your chest, and the rays of stars entering your Bai hui point (Figure 5). Continue to visualize that the rays of the stars enter your Bai hui and pass all way through your body to the *Young quan* (Figure 6) points located at the bottom of your feet. Visualize that the rays from the stars are lifting each heel as you move forward and place each foot on the ground in front of you. When you finish the walk, swallow saliva and visualize it flowing down your esophagus to your lower dan tian area to help condense qi there.

When Driving

It is easy for your body to become tired and stiff from spending too much time in a car every day. The following exercises will help keep qi flowing in your body even though you are in an area of restricted movement. Remember these exercises are to be done in a stopped or parked car so as not to interfere with your driving. Try to be aware that even though you are not able to move your

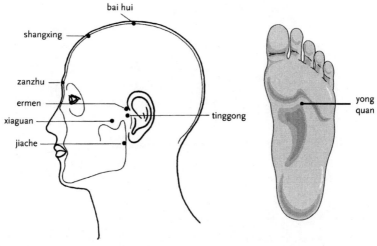

bai hui

shangxing

zanzhu

ermen

xiaguan

jiache

tinggong

yong
quan

Figure 5

Figure 6

body that qi still flows. When you do the movements, keep your mind at the area you are moving.

Gently move your head in a clockwise circle and then gently reverse the direction. As you do this, tell your head to relax. The number of times you do this depends on your situation. Then roll your shoulders forward and then backward and tell them to relax. This will help relieve neck and shoulder stress. Next move your waist and buttocks in a clockwise circle then reverse direction and tell them to relax. This helps qi flow through the *Wei lu* point located in the tail bone area. Knock you teeth together and tell them to relax. After knocking your teeth, massage your gums by circling you tongue inside and outside the gums—first clockwise and then counterclockwise—in a relaxed way. As you do this saliva will collect in your mouth. Gently swallow it and trace its path in your mind to the lower dan tian to help gather qi in this area. While driving, always keep a little awareness in your heart.

Interacting with People

According to qigong and Chinese medical theory, too much talking can drain qi from your body. In your daily interactions with other people try to pay attention to the amount of small talk in which you engage. Many times we engage in such talk so as to be polite, but this can be draining. If you find yourself trapped in a situation that you cannot get out of take the opportunity to practice qigong. At these times, try to focus inward and do the following.

Depending on whether you are sitting or standing, hold your hands, laying your right hand on top of the left palm at your lower dan tian area; tell your body, part by part, to relax. If you have your menses or if you are pregnant, allow your hands to remain at your sides and simply relax your body and mind. In this way, subconsciously you are telling your body that you are keeping your qi inside your body.

Stand slightly on your toes and hold this posture, simply relaxing your mind and body as long as you can. This act will benefit your heart. Before you walk away, swallow some saliva and visualize it going to the dan tian.

If you are seated in an audience, try moving your ankles one at a time in a clockwise circle and then reverse the direction. The number of times you do this should depend on your situation. This will help qi from stagnating in your legs as you sit. You can also massage some acupoints on your hands, fingers, and wrists, such as *Nei guan* (three fingers down from the bottom of your palm in the middle of your forearm), *He gu* (located on the back of your hand between the thumb and index finger). There are many points on our hands that are related to our organs. If you do not know many points, simply massage your hands part by part. You may also choose to simply lay your palms on your legs and turn your focus inside yourself, on your heart, or imagine that your whole body is an empty shell. To end the form before you stand up, simply swallow saliva to your lower dan tian.

While Enjoying Looking at Something

The joy of a pleasant scene—green plants or beautiful flowers—can bring positive qi to your body during this experience. When you are enjoying looking at them, you can visualize sending qi to the back of your head while breathing in. Feel it for a few seconds and then simply exhale through your mouth and think of nothing. Before you walk away, allow saliva to collect in your mouth and gently swallow it. With your mind, trace its path to the dan tian. You may do this as often as you wish while you are in this situation.

Before You Go to Bed

Sit cross-legged on your bed if it is not too soft (or anywhere you are comfortable). If you have to sit on a chair, then keep your feet at shoulders' width. Let go of all the thoughts from your mind. Slowly and gently breathe in through your nose and breathe out through your mouth three times. Each breath thoroughly sends qi into and out of the dan tian. Massage one foot and then the other by using the palm of your hand, not the fingers (especially not the middle finger alone), and make clockwise circles the bottom of your foot. Try to keep the pressure firm but gentle as you do this. Repeat this circular motion for at least 89 times. Your feet have many acupoints related to the various organs; massaging them can relax the mind and promote circulation.

When you are going to sleep, lay on your right side with your right leg straight and relaxed and your left leg slightly bent on top of your right leg. Place the middle finger of your left hand about one hand distance below the hip of the top leg where the Huan tiao acupoint is. Place your right hand under your head so that your thumb and index finger is under your ear. In this way, the qi will focus on circulating along the main channels and go to the lower dan tian.

MEDITATION

Meditation is a still qigong practice and has many styles and levels. There are meditations that are practiced sitting, lying down, and standing. Before you do meditation, you should have some knowledge about it. In its most basic sense, meditation is an exercise that can help you become self-aware. One most common method is that you focus your mind on one thought and forget the outside world while remaining still and quiet. The elementary levels of meditation help to ease and relax the mind. Many meditations focus on mind work or chants. Basically, the purpose of meditation is to let the mind focus gently on one thing. Eventually this can help you enter a carefree state. There are about one hundred styles of meditations that have been passed down through the ages. Each was designed by the sages to will help you achieve this carefree state.

If you are not familiar with meditation you may think that meditation is simply the act of emptying your mind. This is not true. No one can truly empty her (or his) mind. As you meditate, thoughts will come into your mind; this is normal. Do not force out these thoughts. Instead, address these thoughts in a gentle way and let them pass. Just as you should not force thoughts out of your mind, you should not dwell on them either. Take time, try to make the space between the thoughts longer.

Sitting Meditation

From my own experience, the best posture that accommodates both the beginner and advanced practitioner is sitting. A beginner can use a chair if desired: Sit on the front third of the chair; so that your back is away from the back of the chair. If sitting on floor, the basic and better position is to sit on a pad or pillow with your legs crossed with either one or both of your feet resting on top of your knees.

Before meditating, you may eat a little, but it is better to meditate on an empty stomach. This depends on your own health condition. While meditating keep away from wind, and keep your neck and knees warm. The room temperature should be comfortable, not too hot or cold. You can listen to rain, soft ocean waves, water dripping, your own breathing, or your own heartbeats. In the beginning your meditation may only last a few minutes; however, as you advance you may meditate for hours. Practicing advanced meditation is the sole way to reach higher levels of qigong practice and to attain Tao, which, of course, leads you to the spiritual path.

You may have many different experiences while you are meditating, sometimes you may notice physical feelings such as a sore back (which indications that you need to correct your posture) or your legs may fall asleep (indicating that you may have some health problems). The position and structure of your body is very important, and your body will tell you when your posture is not good. Pay attention. When you feel the movement of qi, do not guide—leave it alone. By not using your mind to direct your qi, your mind will become smart—much like a cat watching a mouse. The cat moves quietly, cautiously so as not to startle it. It is best to leave the movement alone, but do not fall asleep. Sometimes you may think you "see" something; try to remember that many of our worries and bad premonitions, including even the "good" scenes, can produce illusions. These illusions are imaginations created by your mind. They are not real, so try to ignore them and they will disappear. Remember to maintain a peaceful and calm mind. Remain aware that you are learning. Remember firmly that you are your own boss, your own Buddha. With this attitude, you will have no trouble. When you have completed your meditation, do not forget to gather the qi back to the lower dan tian—simply swallow some saliva and, with your mind, bring qi back to the lower dan tian and condense it into an egg-yolk-sized ball. Then enter back into the world slowly. If you have menses, simply think of your heart for a minute then get up. This is the beginning of success.

Standing Meditation

Different rules apply to standing meditation than to sitting meditation. There are many types of standing meditation, and each type must be directed by an experienced teacher. Usually, standing meditation should be practiced for no more than an hour per day. During this practice, you may experience spontaneous movement (e.g., twitches, muscle spasms, cramps, etc.). The movements will vary among individuals because of different health conditions; this is normal. When you feel your body change, do nothing. When you feel the qi move, let it flow; do not try to force the movement, do not try to direct it, but be gently aware of the movement. Spontaneous movements that happen during standing meditation are a cleansing process. Be careful, though: Long-time spontaneous movement can drain your qi. Therefore, if you force spontaneous movements, you will cause harm to yourself. Relax your body and mind, and let your body cleanse itself. Eventually, your body will become still after the major qi blockages are removed.

Remember to maintain a peaceful and calm mind and remain aware that you are always learning. Remember firmly that you are your own boss, your own Buddha.

When you have completed your meditation, do not forget to gather the qi back to the lower dan tian. Condense the qi ball with your mind, and then enter back into the world slowly. In the book of *Soaring Crane Qigong*, there is more detail about standing meditation. I do not encourage a beginner to practice this form by herself. Even learning from a teacher, it is good to be knowledgeable about this practice.

Lying Down Meditation

Lying down meditation is relaxing and promotes qi and blood circulation because lying posture makes it easier for the body to relax. You can practice lying meditation for hours without falling asleep. Lying down meditation can be practiced anytime and is good to do before going to sleep or before getting up.

The next grouping of qigong short forms are aimed at helping a specific problem. You will see that some of these forms help to improve such things as vision, skin condition, memory, and breast health, while other forms target specific disorders such as menopause, depression, mouth sores and menstrual problems. I hope that as you read through these forms that you can find something that will help you regulate a problem that you may be experiencing.

Skin Condition

In ancient times some Chinese qigong practitioners used also their own saliva as massage oil to condition their facial skin. In today's society this practice may not sound appealing to you. While you should note that this practice can be done without the saliva part, if you are daring and care to try, here is what you need to do.

In the morning, sit in a cross-legged position and let the thoughts flow from your mind. Rub your hands together palm to palm vigorously until they are hot. Rub your hot hands over your face in an up and down motion as if you were washing your face for a minute or two or as long as you wish. Rub you hands together again until they are hot, this time spit your own saliva into your hands and rub over your face as before for another minute. To practice this massage without using saliva, just repeat the first part. This massage will promote qi flow. The nutria in your saliva will make the skin on your face soft and smooth.

For Vision

There has been much evidence accumulated through years of study in China that qigong practice can help to improve your vision. The following form, by Master Lu Jing-tang was recorded in the *Chinese Qigong Science* magazine. This form helps you learn how to absorb qi, which, in turn, will help improve your vision.

Stand with your heels together, toes slightly separated so that they are approximately four fingers distance apart. Bend your knees slightly, and sink your weight so that it feels like the weight of your body sinks through to the bottom of your feet. Correct your posture so that your back is straight, your chin is slightly tucked in, and your head is held straight. Touch your tongue to the roof of your mouth and gently close your eyes. Slightly tighten your buttocks, and place your hands on your waist. Relax your waist. Breathe naturally until you are relaxed. Slowly move your hands down to your sides, your palms facing slightly backward with your middle fingers on both hands kept straight. Do not allow your hands to contact your body. Focus your mind to the bottom of your feet. As you do this you may get the sensation that your arms are being lifted away. Remain in this posture in a relaxed state for five minutes. As you practice this form regularly, gradually extend the time you stand so that you reach 15 minutes. Once you have achieved 15 minutes, gradually work your way to 30 minutes. At first you might experience hot or cold sensations in your body; this is normal. If you ignore these sensations they will go away as you practice.

During your practice of this form, try to keep your mind vaguely focused on the bottom of your feet. If thoughts come, let them—then let them pass. Each time, try to make the space between thoughts longer so as not to clutter your mind.

When your time is up, remain in the standing position with eyes closed and concentrate on sending the qi to your eyes. Slowly move your eyes in big circles—you can do this one with eyes closed or opened—counterclockwise 36 times, then clockwise 36 times. When you complete this, slowly open your eyes and, keeping your head still, look from side to side as far as you can, then up and down as far as you can. Do each movement 36 times. Next, close your eyes and relax to feel it gently until you feel qi in your eyes. Now, close your eyes tightly, and then open as wide as you can. Repeat seven times. When you have completed this form, slowly stand up and begin to move around normally. This form may also help with some fertility problems in women. It is also used for longevity.

REMOVING A SLIGHT CORNEAL OPACITY (CATARACT). According to Chinese medicine, cataracts are caused by kidney and liver deficiencies, which harm the qi and trap heat inside. To treat it, when you get up in the morning, sit to meditate for a while. With your eyes closed, turn your eyeballs in large circles fourteen times. Then close your eyes tightly for a short while, and suddenly open them wide. Repeat a few times. By persistently doing this exercise for a long time, all types of nebula will be healed. During this period, it is better to not read small print or to have much intercourse as intercourse relates to the kidneys.

To Promote Good Breast Health

This exercise originates from an ancient practice. Sit quietly either cross-legged or in a chair. Try to let your thoughts gently flow from your mind. Keep your mind gently at *Shan zhong* point (inside directly between your nipples). You may sit like this as long as you wish. When you are ready gently cup your right breast with your left hand, slightly touching or without touching, and move your breast in a circular fashion counterclockwise 54 times. Then reverse direction for another 54 times. When you are finished gently release your breast, and do the same movement to your left breast using your right hand and release it gently.

Using your thumb and index finger of your right hand gently pull your left nipple. You should not pull so hard so that you feel discomfort. Then push the nipple inward until it disappears into the mamma. Repeat this 81 times, then switch hands and do the other breast the same way 81 times.

Using your left thumb and index finger to massage your left nipple and your right thumb and index finger to massage your right nipple, gently roll your nipples between your fingers 81 times. When you complete this, cup your breasts in your hands, cupping your left breast with your left hand and your right breast with your right hand. Using a grabbing motion gently massage both breasts at the same time for 81 repetitions. When you have finished sit quietly for a minute or two and focus back to the Shan zhong point. This practice can be done daily or weekly.

Improving Memory

In China, there have been numerous studies performed by doctors and researchers dealing with qigong practice and memory. In cooperation with qigong masters and patients, they have found conclusive evidence that qigong practice can help improve your memory. The following exercise can help you improve your memory by massage and stimulation of certain acupoints of the head.

First we must address the acupoints that will be used in this exercise. You may refer to the drawing to help you get a better idea of their location. (Figure 7) They are *Bai hui, Xin hui, Hou ding, Shuang gu tu, Er chui, Tai yang xu.* You may wish to practice locating these points first so that you are comfortable finding them before continuing the exercise.

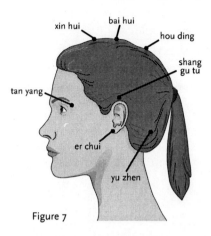

Figure 7

Sit quietly and comfortably either cross-legged or in a chair with your feet as wide as your shoulders. Using the fingers of both hands gently massage in a circular fashion each point for a few seconds. Your mind is gently following your movements. Start at Bai hui. To find this point, with your thumbs touching the top of your ears, touch your middle fingers at the top of your head—where they meet is the Bai hui point. Then move to the Xin hui. Move the fingers to the back of the head to Hou ding and very gently massage this point with no pressure for a few seconds. Next move your fingers to the point called Shuang gu tu again gently massage this point for a few seconds then move on to the Er chui points on the earlobes. Continue to the point, Tai yang, located at the hollowed area on your temples. Return to the front of your head to Xin hui, and then finally back to Bai hui. Repeat this sequence ten times. The massage should be very gentle.

When you have finished the massage, sit quietly and slowly close your eyes. Keep your tongue on the roof of your mouth behind your teeth, and focus your mind to the Bai hui point.

Another practice for improving memory is to guide the qi back and forth: from the top of your head, Bai hui, down the middle channel to the prinium, Hui yin. Sit quietly and slowly close your eyes. Place your tongue on the roof of your mouth behind your teeth, and focus your mind to the Bai hui point. Visualize absorbing qi from the universe; it is streaming into your Bai hui point. Gently use your mind to visualize the qi slowly flowing from your Bai hui point to your throat. Let the qi continue to flow along the middle channel to the lower dan tian to your Hui yin point, which is located in the region between your vagina and anus. As the qi approaches the Hui yin point, very gently contract your vagina and anus. Once the qi has reached your Hui yin point, use your mind to slowly bring the qi up again to your Bai hui point. Once the qi has passed your anus, you can relax that area. (The qi can leak out a body orifice if it is not closed as the qi passes.) Repeat this cycle 10 times.

As you practice this exercise your breathing must be soft, gentle, and deep but without force. When you finish, lay your two palms at the lower dan tian area with the right palm over the left, and sit quietly for a few moments. When you are finished, slowly open your eyes and get up.

A third exercise that you can do is to visualize a sun the size of an egg-yolk sitting in your lower dan tian area. Imagine that the sun is floating on the water, because a qi ball should not be still. Your mouth should be closed, and your tongue should naturally touch the roof of your mouth. Try to keep this visualization for 15 to 20 minutes. Then swallow some saliva, and you are done.

Sleeping Disorder

Any relaxation type of qigong can help improve sleeping problems. If you are going through menopause or are having trouble sleeping try this exercise in the evening.

Form your left hand into an empty fist so that you can see the hollow. Bring your fist around to your back to your *Ming men* point located between your kidneys and above your sacrum. Using the fist to massage the Ming men point making counterclockwise circles 108 times. When you finish, repeat the exercise using the right fist. Ming men is where the original qi is tied and is the home of jing. This practice will bring your scattered qi and shen back so that you can sleep normally.

Left Brain, Right Brain

The Yellow Emperor's *Nei Jing* points out that when a person's brain is properly functioning and in good condition the aging process will slow down. The following exercises split the brain into left and right segments, conditioning the right and left brain segments respectively.

TO HELP RIGHT BRAIN FUNCTIONS. Close your left hand into a tight fist then relax it and repeat this movement 300 times. When you completed this, start with the thumb and fold your fingers into your palm one at a time to create a fist. When you have made the fist, straighten your fingers one at a time starting with your little finger until your hand is open. Repeat 100 times.

During the day when you have free time, visualize objects in your mind and try to move them around or alter their shapes and sizes. Try to make these images as sharp and clear as you can. Once you have accomplished this, try adding color and texture to the image as well.

TO HELP CONDITION THE LEFT BRAIN. Take a few minutes to think of a process that is familiar to you. Once you have gone through the process in your mind, reverse it and see if you can do the process step-by-step backwards. Also, try reading a few paragraphs backwards or reciting a sentence backwards.

After completing these exercises rub your hands together until they are hot. Then place your hands on the back of your head at the base of your skull so as to cover the *Yu zhen* points, which are located at the base of your skull. Try to let thoughts flow through your mind and keep your hands there for three minutes. When time is up, you may return to the day at hand.

Menopause

Qigong is very effective in helping with problems caused by menopause. Because of my qigong practice, I was able to go through my menopause peacefully and quickly. I did not experience any of the classic symptoms such as sweating and uneasiness. I slept well and had as much energy as I usually do.

As a woman goes through menopause, the hormonal changes occurring in her body might normally cause mood swings and physical sensations (as we all know). The following qigong exercise is designed to help a woman go through menopausal changes in her life.

This form can be performed standing, sitting, or lying down. Choose the starting posture that you prefer.

❖ If standing, stand with your feet as wide as your shoulders and with
   your knees slightly bent. Be sure that you have good straight posture
   with your arms resting softly at your sides.

❖ If sitting sit comfortably in the front third of a chair so that your back is straight, your feet are flat on the floor, and your hands rest palms down on your thighs.

❖ If lying down, lie on your back with your feet as wide as your shoulders and with your arms at your sides. Be sure that the tip of your tongue is placed on the roof of your mouth just behind your teeth before you begin.

Once you are in the starting position of your choice, relax your body and breathe softly and slowly in and out through your nose. Try to let thoughts pass through your mind so as not to fixate on any one thought. When you are ready, visualize that there are four lines touching your body. Two of the lines are on either side of your body extending from the top of your head, following the side of your body to the bottom of your feet. The other two follow the front and back of your body and again extend from the top of your head to the bottom of your feet. Once you visualize these lines, use your mind to relax each body part that the lines would touch. Start at the top of your head and continue to the bottom of your feet. This process is done one line at a time, but the order of the lines is not important.

Let us walk through this process so that you get the idea. I will select the line touching the right side of your body first. Visualize that there is an imaginary line touching the right side of your body that starts at the top of your head and ends at the bottom of your feet. Breathe with soft, regular inhalations and exhalations. Beginning at the Bai hui point at the top of your head try to relax that area. Slowly and gently trace the line to the side of your head and relax that area. Move to the side of your neck and relax it. Move to your right shoulder and relax it. Continue down the arm to your fingers and relax the entire arm, hand and fingers. Finish down the side of your leg, past the knee and ankle to the feet. Continue to relax each part as you come to it. When you have completed this, move on to the other three lines. Repeat this entire sequence two more times so that you have relaxed each line three times. When you have completed the exercise, try to concentrate on your lower dan tian for a few minutes, and then slowly open your eyes to bring yourself back into your surroundings. As always, if you have your menses at the time simply keep your mind at your heart for a minute or just relax, instead of focusing on your lower dan tian.

If you prefer, you can visualize milky-white colored water flowing over your body rather than lines touching your body. The process would be the same as described above except that you would relax the part of your body over which the water flowed. When you have completed this three times finish the exercise as mentioned above.

Amenorrhoea

Amenorrhoea is a condition in which menses stops completely before the woman goes through menopause. It is usually caused either by extreme physical exertion, extreme emotional disturbances, or other extreme conditions that result in the body harboring too much cold or yin energy. The type of qigong that helps correct this condition is called Strengthening Gong, which helps release extremes and helps in the absorption of yang energy. This exercise can be done either sitting or standing, and you can alternate positions each time you practice this exercise.

I would like to first address the breathing in this form because it is different than what we have been discussing up to this point. All of the exercises we have discussed so far allow you to breathe naturally or inhale and exhale deeply while doing the exercise. When practicing this form, be sure to pull in your abdomen when you inhale and push out your abdomen when you exhale. This way of breathing massages and exercises your ovaries as you breathe.

Keep your mind vaguely focused at the lower dan tian. Practice this exercise 15 to 20 minutes, two to three times a day until your menses comes. If your menses comes but the flow is less than normal, focus your mind a little more at the lower dan tian. If the flow is more than normal, then reduce your mind work at your lower dan tian. If your menses is very heavy, then focus your attention to your Shan zhong point. You need to adjust this according to your own body type.

In addition to Strengthening Gong, you may also practice the following exercise. You can either sit or stand to do this. Rub your palms together until they are hot. Then place your palms over your ovaries and massage them in a circular fashion. Massage by making 54 counterclockwise circles followed by 54 clockwise circles. Daily practice of this exercise can help menses return. This exercise helps qi to remove the blockages in your abdomen to speed up healing.

Abnormal Menses

If your menses is abnormal in that you only flow a little, you may have a deficiency. You can practice sitting meditation, vaguely keeping your mind at your lower dan tian. Breathe naturally. Meditate for 30 to 40 minutes, three to four times daily. After your normal menses comes, reduce the exercise to one to two times daily. After your menses returns to normal, turn your mind to your Shan zhong point instead of your dan tian. Chinese herbal formulas are very effective for any type of abnormal menses, and they will speed up your healing when you practice qigong at the same time. (See Chapter 7.)

During Pregnancy

A pregnant mother's physical and emotional state can directly affect the physical and emotional states of her unborn child. If you are pregnant, it is extremely important that you keep yourself as balanced physically and emotionally as you possibly can. An unborn baby's emotional state is very fragile and if disturbed it can seriously affect the baby's health and energy balance. According to Taoism, when a fetus is formed by semen and egg, the primary qi is born with the fetus. That primary qi is called "pure yang qi," which is not polluted. After conception but before birth, the baby can become polluted by the mother's emotional disturbances, such as a sudden shock, fear, or grief. In the Chinese culture great care is taken to keep a pregnant woman away from situations that can bring about extreme emotions. Self-cultivation includes the knowledge of eating the right foods and herbs to help the pregnant women retain emotional and physical balance and prevent the fetus from illness. Following are some qigong exercises that can help you keep balanced during your pregnancy. A form that suits all pregnant women is meditation in a relaxed state with your mind empty of distractions and focused vaguely at your Shan zhong point.

Vomiting During Pregnancy

The causes of vomiting during pregnancy can vary. I will include such discussions in this book. If you have problems with morning sickness or vomiting any time during your pregnancy, try this short form to help alleviate these symptoms.

Stand with your feet parallel, a little wider than your shoulders, and be sure to have good straight posture. Tuck your chin slightly so that your neck and head are in line with your back, and place your tongue to the roof of your mouth behind your teeth. Lace your fingers in front of your chest, palms facing up, but not touching your chest. Relax your shoulders. Exhale slowly while separating your hands and letting them fall slowly to the sides of your body. At the same time that you lower your arms and exhale, bend your knees slightly at about 70 degrees so that your buttocks sink. Your breathing should remain natural throughout this exercise. Hold this posture for ten seconds, breathing naturally. Inhale, slowly stand up, and bring your hands up to the beginning posture (laced in front of your chest). Once you are standing up, allow your breathing to return to normal. Repeat five times. When you have completed five repetitions, begin again but sink lower this time so that you bend your knees a little deeper, approximately one and a half feet from the ground. Repeat this five times. When you have finished, repeat the sequence again by bending your knees as far as they can so that your hands either rest on the floor or come as close to it as you can. Hold this position for ten seconds, and repeat the sequence five times. To end the form, stand up for the last time. Close your eyes, and allow your breathing to return to normal. When this happens, slowly open you eyes and go about your day as usual. Gently keep your mind on breathing and movements.

Lower Abdominal Pain and Frequent Urination

If you suffer from lower abdominal pain and frequent urination, practice of the following exercise can help to alleviate your discomfort. Lie on your back, and bend your knees so that your heels are as close to your buttocks as you can get them. Lay your hands on your knees or thighs, whichever you can best reach. Inhale slowly through your mouth, and send the breath to the lower abdomen until it is full. Exhale slowly through your nose, and, as you do so, gently contract your reproductive and anal areas. Repeat seven times. When you have finished, get up slowly and continue with your normal daily routine.

Lying Down Meditation for the Prevention
of Illness and Longevity

This particular exercise is used to prevent illness and increase your longevity. Results are best obtained if this exercise is practiced early in the morning or at least right after you awake from a night sleep. You may choose one from the following.

1. Lie on your back and place a pillow under your neck to help support it. The pillow should keep your head and neck even with your spine. Place your arms at your sides, palms down and a thumb-length away from your body. You may close your eyes or keep them half closed. Your mouth should be closed and your tongue should naturally touch the roof of your mouth. Your feet should be a little bit closer than shoulder-width. Relax and begin to breathe slowly and steadily. Think of nothing; just listen to and count your breaths. One cycle of inhalation and exhalation will equal one repetition. Repeat 360 times. As you practice this exercise, you may begin to feel a separation sensation in your bones and joints and your body may feel as if it were in the clouds; this is a normal experience for this exercise. When it is time to end, you move your attention at the lower dan tian, swallow some saliva, and trace its path to the lower dan tian. Then rub your hands together until hot, and massage your face.

2. Lie in the same way as the above. Place your arms at the sides of your body. Your palms should be down and about a thumb's length away from your body. Keep your feet approximately one foot apart. Let your thoughts flow from your mind, and allow yourself to think of nothing. Slowly and gently inhale through your nose visualize that you are inhaling qi from the universe and sending the qi with your breath to the lower dan tian. Create the image in your mind that the qi you are inhaling is cleansing your organs as it travels to the lower dan tian. Exhale slowly through your mouth and let the breath come from the lower dan tian. Visualize that you are releasing all that you cleansed from your organs. You can continue the cleansing breath as long as you wish. When you are finished, turn on to your right side. Allow your natural breathing to return, concentrate on the lower dan tian, and condense your qi into a tiny ball. When you are finished, rise slowly and return to your daily routine.

   As you continue to practice this exercise, you may experience a gurgling noise in your lower abdomen; this is normal and is a signal to you that you are successfully practicing the exercise.

   If you have menses, stop doing the visualization; just rest and relax.

3. Qigong uses imagery created in the mind to help manifest those images in reality. You can use those images to sculpt yourself into the person that you want to become. You can use the following format to create the setting for the visualization that best suits what you would like to balance. For example, if you wish to become a more polite and gentle person, you need to balance your aggressive energy for your

own health as well as how you affect others. Try the following. Lie on your back, and place you arms at you sides, palms down about a thumb's distance away from your body. Inhale slowly and softly through your nose, and exhale in the same way through your mouth. At the same time, picture yourself being a very polite and gentle person. Practicing this type of imagery in a qigong state can help you to balance the yin and yang energies and harmonize them inside your body.

4. Lie on your back with your head on a flat pillow, and elevate your feet slightly with a pillow, folded blanket, or whatever you have. Cover yourself so that you are warm and comfortable. Place your arms at the sides of your body, palms down, and touch your tongue to the roof of your mouth directly behind your teeth. Exhale through your mouth three times in succession to release stagnant qi from your body. As you do this, saliva should collect in your mouth. Use the saliva to rinse your mouth. Swallow it, tracing its path down your throat to your lower dan tian. Repeat the exhalation and saliva-swallowing three times. Allow your body to relax, and listen to your heart beating. Forget that the world exists. Try to allow yourself to forget that even your body exists. You may do this as long as you wish.

As you practice this exercise regularly, you may begin to feel a sweaty sensation on the palms of your hands; this in good. Once you experience this sensation, change the position of your hands to loose fists, and continue to practice as described above. Practicing with your hands open helps to unlock your qi channels and discharge the sick qi.

To end this practice, bring your thoughts to the lower dan tian, and focus you mind there for a minute. You may at the same time swallow some saliva and trace it to the lower dan tian.

5. The following qigong can be practiced to help promote healing. If you are ill or recovering from an injury, practice of this form can facilitate your recovery. Before you begin, first comb your hair with a wooden comb (made of peach, date, or horn of ox or cow—they have some healing function) or simply with your fingers so that your scalp becomes relaxed and the circulation is promoted. Allow your hair to fall naturally. Then lie on your back without a pillow and with your feet apart slightly less than shoulder-width. Place your arms at your sides, palms down. Allow your thoughts to pass through your mind, and relax. When you are ready, inhale through your nose, and then gently hold your breath as long as you can. While you are holding your breath, try to concentrate on the area of your body that is injured or ill. This will help the healing process by moving qi to that area. When you cannot hold your breath any longer, exhale slowly and allow your breathing to return to normal. When you are ready, inhale slowly and repeat the exercise. Do this a total of ten times. Do not practice this if you are sleepy, because you might fall asleep. End the form as indicated above.

When you begin to gain weight, your inner system is no longer in balance. Qigong practice can help heal this system by putting your body back in balance and helping to facilitate the weight loss process. Once you have lost the weight, qigong practice will help keep your internal structure in balance. When practicing qigong to help you to lose weight, it is a good idea to practice on an empty stomach. In order for our bodies to metabolize consumed foods, it requires energy. When we practice qigong, we become more aware of our bodies' own internal energy. By practicing qigong regularly, you can assist your body in raising your metabolic rate. Though practice of any qigong form can assist you when you are trying to lose weight, there are forms that exist that specifically were designed to help the weight loss process. Remember that practicing this form will not magically make you lose the weight you desire. As with any form of qigong exercise, you must eat sensibly, drink enough water, and get proper rest so that your body can become properly balanced. If you are following the aforementioned guidelines to lose extra weight, try the following qigong exercise.

Lie on your back with your arms at your sides, palms down, and a little away from your body. Slowly close your eyes, and place your tongue to the roof of your mouth directly behind your teeth. Move your tongue around your upper and lower gums in a clockwise fashion. This will cause saliva to collect in your mouth. Rinse your mouth with it slowly like you would rinse your mouth when you brush your teeth. Swallow it little bits at a time. As you swallow your saliva, trace its path with your mind: down your esophagus to your lower dan tian. Imagine it warming the dan tian area as it reaches its destination.

Inhale softly through your nose as deeply as you can, and then exhale through your mouth as much as you can. When you inhale again, inhale in five short, successive breaths through your nose and without exhaling so that your lungs are full. When you have inhaled to your maximum, gently contract your genital area and anus and swallow your saliva. As before, trace with your mind the path from your throat to the lower dan tian. Then exhale thoroughly through your mouth. Remember to keep these inhalations and exhalations soft and gentle and not forceful. If during the inhalation process you need to exhale, do so just enough for you to continue the inhalation—do not exhale thoroughly at this time. The idea here is to take more inhalations than exhalations. You may do this daily before a meal for a half-hour or longer. As you practice this exercise, try to increase the number of inhalations you take before you exhale thoroughly. When you finish the exercise, have some rice soup.

After practicing for a time, you may have a better appetite, digest well, and be more energetic. After a long time, practitioners do not eat as much as they did before, yet they retain a normal weight and get enough nutrition because they are not draining qi. Instead, they are able to gather more nutrition because they have mastered the skill of absorbing qi.

Depression

We all have times in our lives when we feel depressed. Sometimes we dwell in our problems, thinking about them constantly. We do not give ourselves a break, no matter how large or small the problems are. No matter how difficult the situation may be, you must take care of yourself. If you let a situation consume you, it will disturb your physical well-being and manifest even more problems. If you take a short time out of your day to do something for yourself, you will see that you will be able to tend to your problems with a fresh mind. The following qigong can help to lighten your heart when you face situations that get you down.

Sit in a comfortable chair with good posture and your feet flat on the floor. Place your hands palms down on your thighs and keep your head lifted, but hold your chin inward slightly. Place the tip of your tongue to the roof of your mouth directly behind your teeth. Breathe softly and slowly, inhaling through your nose and exhaling gently through your mouth.

With your mind, look inside your body; visualize that there are no organs and bones, just an empty shell. Picture a sun setting with a reddish glow where your heart should be. Focus your attention gently on the sun so that your problems are out of your sight. Just continue to sit and enjoy the glow from the sunset breathing softly and slowly. You may stay in this state as long and as often as you like. If you are pressed for time or have difficulty sitting still, try five minutes at a time. When you are ready, visualize that your organs have returned and are functioning well. Think of your heart for a minute and knock your teeth together while doing so. When saliva collects in your mouth, swallow it and visualize it sending nourishing energy to your lower dan tian. Slowly open your eyes, and return to your daily routine.

Another exercise is to lie on your left side, relax first, breathe in through your mouth, and exhale through your nose. Remain this way for 20 minutes or longer, depending on your situation.

For Longevity and Treating Sterility

These practices are chosen from *The Causes of Diseases* written by a well-known physician-qigong master, Chao Yuan-fang (A.D. 581–618). You can do one or all of them. Each one helps preserve longevity and treat sterility. Acupuncture and herbal formulas are also good for such problems and will assist in speeding up the healing.

FORM A. After the sun sets and when the moon comes out, face the moon and stand, relaxed. Hold your breath until you can no longer hold it, and then breathe out softly and slowly. Repeat this eight times. Then lift up your chin, and swallow the moonlight (like a fish in the water). Swallow the saliva slowly. Practice this for as long as you like. This practice also benefits the brain and mind.

FORM B. Massage the kidneys before going to bed. Facing the north, sit to relax with your eyes closed for a while. Then with your mind's eye, look at the top of your head. Touch your tongue to the roof of your mouth, and slightly contract your private parts. Now gently massage the kidney spots, 120 circles or more—and the more, the better. Then you can sleep.

FORM C. Assume the standing posture, feet as wide as your shoulders. Relax. Form your hands into two empty fists, and use the tiger mouth points (the hollows) to gently knock the two kidney spots 108 times. When knocking softly, the movement should penetrate the energy into the kidneys in depth. Breathe naturally.

For Treating Numbness Caused by Cold, Wind, or Dampness

This is from an ancient book by Immortal Chen. The steps are:

1. Sit on the floor, put your right heel on your left big toe and hold it backward. Inhale through your nose and exhale through your mouth in a natural, slow way. Hold your toe position as long as you wish. Then exchange; your left heel is on the right toe. You can also hold the top of one foot, touching the opposite knee. Do this alternatively with each foot.

2. Lie on the floor or a hard bed with your feet apart but your knees touching each other. Stretch your back, then inhale through your mouth slowly until your abdomen sticks out full of qi. Exhale through your mouth again. Do this seven times.

3. Lie on your back with your legs and arms straight. Inhale softly and thoroughly, and then exhale slowly. Repeat seven times. Then lift up your lower body and move in circles: 30 circles counterclockwise, then 30 circles clockwise.

4. Lie on the floor on your stomach. Cross your fingers; your arms and your hands push to press on the floor. Stretch your head and back backward, and inhale and exhale softly. Repeat five times.

5. Assume standing posture, lift your toes up, inhale and exhale. Repeat five times.

6. Lie on your back with your arms and legs straight. Keep your heels outward with your toes facing each other. Inhale slowly, softly and thoroughly, then exhale slowly. Repeat seven times.

For Treating Cold and Preventing Flu

1. When you begin to catch a cold, visualize that your heart is like a fireball. The reddish flames spread all over your body and burn the germs. Repeat until the cold is driven out. End the form by keep your mind at the lower dan tian for a minute.

2. When there is flu spreading, you visualize there is a reddish, shiny fireball near your heart. You may also steam some strong, dark vinegar inside the room and inhale it. It kills the virus in the air and in your breathing system. You can also get some Chinese herbal formulas such as Ban lan gen. Take it for three to five days. There are more tips for using herbs for treating colds in my upcoming *Herbal Food* book.

TRANSLATIONS

For treating acute sickness
— Gao Lian

Suddenly you feel sick,
If you ignore it, it will harm you later,
So you restrain your mind and go to your bedroom,
Take off your clothes and lie in a warm bed,
Form empty fists and you lay them on the sides.
With the incenses* burning,
You knock your teeth,
Then swallow 36 times your saliva,

Now that your lower dan tian has gathered more qi.
Your mind guides the qi to any part of the body,
Of course now the best spot should be where the sickness is.
Doing so until you get sweaty,
And then you can stop.
Help you more than to pray for a cure,
Will this practice be."

*The Chinese incenses are made of herbs that can kill some germs in the air.

THE SIX-EXHALING SOUNDS EXERCISE. The Six Exhaling Sounds Exercise was first taught by a great Taoist physician, Tao Hon-jing (A.D. 452–536). It was made popular by another great Taoist physician, the King of Medicine, Sun Si-miao (A.D. 581–682). Some masters also add some simple movements to this form to assist this exhalation. This practice was developed to help cleanse and nourish the organs. As the name of the exercise indicates, there are six sounds that will be used. Each one relates to a specific major organ. The six sounds are: *her-* ("kher") this sound is related to the heart; *hu-* ("hoo") is related to the spleen; *s-* ("ss") is related to the lungs; *chui-* ("chwee") is related to the kidneys; *xu* ("shu") is related to the liver; and *xi* ("shi-", but the tongue is flat) is related to the three jiao or the visceral cavities surrounding the organs. As you practice this exercise you will exhale each of the above sounds. As you exhale each sound six to 12 times, you will say them softly and slowly and shape your mouth in a particular way to pronounce the sound. As you do this, visualize toxins being cleansed out of the specific organ that you are working on at the time.

This exercise can be practiced in any one of the three postures: sitting, standing, or lying down.

❖ If standing, stand with your feet shoulders with apart and your hands naturally on your sides. Gently touch your middle fingers to the side seams of your pants, and slightly lift your shoulders up.

❖ If you are sitting, sit comfortably in front third of a chair; place your feet flat on the floor about one foot apart, and place your hands, palms down, on your knees.

❖ If lying down, lie on your back with your arms at your sides about one thumb's distance away from your body, and keep your feet about a foot apart. Be sure you do not fall asleep.

To begin, choose one of the above positions. Once you are comfortable, slowly close your eyes and inhale through your nose softly filling the lungs. Then exhale thoroughly, saying the first sound kher softly as long as you can so that the breath is coming up from the bottom of your abdomen. As you exhale the sound, visualize that all toxins are being cleansed from that organ. Repeat this process six to twelve times for each of the six sounds. For a severe illness, you can repeat to 36 times or follow a qigong healer's advice. If you remember the relationship between the Five Elements, you will be able to heal yourself more quickly. I have successfully healed myself of colds and sore throats by using this practice. Remember, do not to use your mind much when exhaling or inhaling. The best way is to exhale so softly that you can barely hear it yourself.

I have translated the "Song of the Six Exhaling" handed down by Sun and the definition by Gao Lian. As you read these you will see that the Chinese used this form as a means of treating different ailments by using a form of sound therapy. You should note when reading this translation that it was written by men for men. That does not mean that it was not applied to women; it is just the historical situation of the time.

"Song of the Six Exhaling"
—Sun Si-miao

(K)her- goes to the heart channel. The illnesses related to this channel
shows the symptom on the tongue. The patient's mouth feels dry
and the tongue looks "rough," also the patient feels heat in the
chest. If the patient feels much heat in the chest, she or he should
open the mouth wider when exhaling. If not such a case, the
mouth should not open wide. They also can do this with the
fingers crossed and stretch the arms above the head when exhaling.
Do more than six times.

Hu- sound relates to the spleen. If her/his sickness is related to this
channel, the symptom is shown in the stomach and abdomen.
They feel bloated, depressed, and maybe with light heat. Exhale
this one with the lips puckered. Do more than six times.

Chui- is related to the kidneys. If her/his abdomen and waist feel cold,
exhale this one to heal. The patient may kneel down level with the
two hands holding the knees and exhale.

Xu- goes to the liver channel. The liver is related to the eyes. If the eyes
are red and sick, the patient exhales the xu-. When exhaling, the
patient can also at the same time open the eyes wide, thinking to
send out the illness of the eyes.

Xi- is related to the three-jiao system. When these areas do not feel
   good, exhale
xi- If there is much heat feeling inside the chest, the patient may lie on
   the side to exhale.
Ss- goes to the lung channel. The problems of nasal and skin are related
   to the lung. If the nasal passages catch cold or feel heat, do this
   one. It also heals the skin ulcer or sore. The patient also may
   stretch the two arms above the head when doing this one, as if the
   hands were holding something heavy."

Defined by Gao Lian:

The first one is the Ss-.
Ss- works magic,
Which is connected with the lung and also the nose,
If one has a consumptive cold or heat, or skin ulcers
He can exhale Ss- to take care of all.
The second is the Kher-.
Heh- is related to the King Heart,
And the symptoms show on the tongue,
The mouth will feel dry and he may feel a smothering sensation
Then one must exhale the heh-,
According to the degree of the sickness,
Then the sickness in the chest
Surely will be cleansed away.
The third is the hu-,
It belongs to the spleen shen that is in charge of the Earth element
The symptom will be a bloated abdomen
With heat and dysphoria,
The four limbs will feel heavy,
Also feel difficult breathing,
So this patient should exhale the hu-
To regulate the qi that will heal.
The fourth is the xu-,
Which goes to the shen of the liver*
The symptom shows in the patient's eyes,
Teary, red, or growing nebula.
Caused by the heat in the liver that has driven the qi upward.
So if the patient exhales the xu-
It will work faster than a formula.
The fifth is the chui-
That goes to the kidneys.
The patient's symptom is poor in hearing,
And his waist feels cold,

His knees feel weak,
And impotence is one of the symptoms.
So softly and long he exhales the chui-,
And there will be no need to seek medicine from the outside.
The sixth is the xi-.
Xi- treats the illnesses in the three-jiao,
When the qi in there is not in harmony,
It will harm the three-jiao.
The patient just exhales the xi- repeatedly
And the qi will be normalized.

I have provided in this chapter qigong exercises that you can incorporate into your daily lives. I hope they help you achieve a more balanced state of existence. Remember, though, that cultivation does not mean qigong practice only—it also includes working on the heart, good eating practices, and the incorporation of traditional Chinese medicine into your life. In the chapters that follow, I wish to introduce you to these topics and provide you with more helpful information.

Chapter 6

Only the fortunate one can enjoy reading valuable books and leave the best treasure to their children.
—*Immortal Lu Dong-bin*

Qigong as a Way of Life

In this chapter, I have compiled eastern thoughts and practices dealing with every day occurrences so that you may see how the principles in this book combine to become what I call cultivation. You may find the concepts foreign to a western way of thinking, and that is fine. Many western concepts were foreign to me when I arrived in this country as well. It is all about learning to understand each other. I have arranged these thoughts alphabetically by subject matter to make the reading easier.

ADVICE FOR MOTHERS

When you are pregnant, try to keep yourself away from situations that may be excessive so as not to disturb the baby; too much or too little of anything may not be good for the baby. Also, do not take drugs or alcohol. Such things can poison the fetus. What you eat is what your baby eats so it is very important to take care of yourself during this time of your life.

If you are pregnant and are planning to breast-feed, eat organic food. Harmful chemicals can cause much damage. Fruits and vegetables are often sprayed with chemicals that when ingested can remain in our systems for years. If they enter your system they will enter your unborn child's system as well. For example, it takes between four to thirty years to totally cleanse your body of the toxin of DDLP (dichlovos) and six to ten years to clean BHC (benzene hexachloride) out of the human system. Both of these chemicals are commonly used in insecticides.

When you are preparing foods, be certain that your fruits and vegetables are clean. If they are organic, they are chemical free, but bacteria can still exist on the outside skin. The Chinese use a combination of dark vinegar, roasted sesame oil, and garlic on salads. Not only does it taste good, but it is believed that this combination can kill harmful bacteria as well. Pregnancy is a delicate time so you want to take all precautions to prevent illness.

If you are pregnant or have just given birth and are between the ages of eighteen and forty-eight years of age, avoid eating too much hot and spicy food during you menstrual period. Hot and spicy foods will cause heat internally and can lead to miscarriages, acute mastitis, and constipation. You should also avoid foods with cold properties; they can cause harm to the stomach and spleen and result in abdominal pain.

Modern researchers have proven that disturbed emotions can affect a fetus. According to ancient Taoism, the primary qi is born with the fetus before the sex is distinguished. Before birth, the baby can be "polluted" by the mother's emotional disturbances. That is why you may hear the Chinese people giving advice to an upset pregnant woman, "For your baby's sake, do not anger yourself." Or, "Please stop crying, or the health of you and your baby will be affected; you might cause an abortion."

During the month after a mother gives birth, it is important that the new mother keep her body warm and dry. According to Chinese medicine, when a woman is giving birth, her joints are completely opened thus it takes a long time for the body to completely recover from this. If during the month after the birth, some dampness or cold attacks her body, it is believed that besides being ill, she will have arthritis in her later years.

A healthy child can cry and be spoiled, but her or his cries will not last a long time. When a young child is fussy most of the time, it is an indication that there must be something wrong with this child's health. Take your child to see an experienced doctor if your child is fussy most of the time.

If a young baby's (a few months old) emotions are disturbed, her or his health can be affected. For example, a loud noise can scare a baby and disturb his or her shen—the mind/heart; this can tangle her qi. As a result, this can cause the child to cry without stopping, to suddenly cry in a dream, or to convulse. An emotional disturbance will cause the color of the child's feces to change; for example, sometimes it is dark green.

If you have consulted an herbal physician for a remedy for your child, the following is a common way to administer it. If it is in powder form, mix the powder with a little water into a thin soup-like consistency in a teaspoon first. Hold the baby face up in your arms at chest level. Put the spoon at one side of the baby's tongue and let the liquid little by little go underneath the tongue, so the child can swallow slowly and not choke. When my children were babies, if they would not swallow the medicine, my mother and I would work together as a team. I would hold the baby and my mother would gently hold the baby's nose and feed the medicine the same way that I described above.

I often see some people holding a baby under the arms with the baby's abdomen exposed in cold weather. It is important to keep a baby's stomach and lower abdomen covered and protected because this is where life starts.

I always think it is a bad idea to let a child sleep alone in the darkness. I remember when I was in elementary school, during the nights when my young brother and I were home alone, my brother would fall asleep quickly because his older sister was next to him. Yet it would take a long time for me to sleep. Any dark shadows moving on the walls and on the windows would give my imagination plenty of fuel. My heart would beat fast, and I would sweat. Even in the hot, humid summer, I often covered my head and fell asleep in fear. Such fears in children can upset the balance of qi in their bodies.

I notice many toddlers still wearing diapers. Just think to yourself: how would you feel if your bottom were covered tight all the time? Train the child to use the potty as soon as the child can walk. Try to let your child use fewer diapers, especially if it is a girl. Use diapers that are cotton and chemical-free. Exposure of the baby's private parts, especially the vagina, to such chemicals can be toxic to her body and can pollute the qi inside.

Chinese parents cook balanced meals for their children, ensuring from the start that the qi within their bodies is balanced.

Chinese mothers often use foods for prevention of illness. For example, when the child is older (two years or older), a common remedy is used in the spring to prevent flu or sore throat. It is a remedy called *Ban lan gen*, an herbal powder made from a plant called Ban lan, given for five days as a prevention.

Additionally, in spring, some mothers feed their babies (between four and twelve months old) a soupspoon of milky juice made from fresh chestnuts to cleanse the child's body. In hot summer, mung bean soup with a little rock sugar is often used so that the child does not overheat. In autumn, eating pears is more beneficial because pears function by releasing hidden heat in the lung; thus, they act as prevention for winter coughing. You can also cook a pear. A popular way of preparing pears is to remove the core, put a small chunk of rock sugar inside and steam it in a bowl. (The Asian pear, round and brown in color, is the best for cooking.) Let the child eat the pear and drink the soup. Even today in China, herbal remedies are more widely used to prevent and cure illness instead of relying on chemical cures.

AGING

A tip for longevity: always remember to lift up the corners of your mouth. By doing so, you keep your kidneys healthy, and, according to qigong and Chinese medical theory, healthy kidneys slow the aging process. Though this claim has never been proven by Western science, there have been experiments in this area in China since ancient times. In addition to qigong practice you can take good care of your kidneys by eating a balanced diet, including foods that benefit the kidneys such as black soybeans, sesame seeds, and raw pine nuts for example. Another prevention for kidney health is moderating your sex life.

IN THE BATHROOM

Bathrooms in China are different than bathrooms in America. In China there are conventional western fixtures but there are also conventional eastern fixtures. The eastern fixture is a squat toilet that allows you to relieve yourself from a squatting position rather that a sitting position. I prefer the squat toilet because it exercises the knees and is cleaner than sitting style. The Chinese believe that sitting on the toilet for a long time is unnatural and can cause hemorrhoids.

Advice from Chinese medical theory is to not read in the bathroom; use the bathroom as it is intended and simply relieve yourself. Holding in urine or a bowel movement for a long time is not good because they are the wastes that your body is discarding. Feces usually contain harmful bacteria, and it is not good for your body to have this stored inside.

When urinating, clench your teeth. This act insures that your essence will not leak from your kidneys.

When you have a bowel movement, form your hands into two empty fists gently and lay them on your knees and keep your mouth closed so that you discharge it quickly and do not drain your energy. If you want to have a faster bowel movement, before you go to the bathroom, squat down like you are doing a deep knee bend. Stay in the squatting position with your weight forward on your toes. At the same time, hold a mouthful of water, and stretch your arms forward at shoulder height. Divide the water into three portions and swallow the first two portions hard and then the third normally.

BREAST MILK

Women's breasts are very delicate, especially when breast-feeding. Care must be taken not to press the breasts in any way during this time. Such action could cause damage to the qi channels in the mammary, thus causing proper circulation of the milk to become blocked and the breast to become red and swollen. The milk from this breast is then considered toxic and, of course, is harmful to the child. This situation can also have later repercussions to the mother as well.

When you need to stop nursing, eat roasted germinated barley. This herb stops the lactating process. It can be purchased in a Chinese herbal store. The clerk there will divide it into portions for you and teach you how to boil it. To take it, you simply boil it in water and drink the resulting tea that this process produces.

If you need to increase the quantity of your breast milk, again germinated barley can help—but it is processed in a different way. If you tell the clerk why you need it, he or she will direct you as to how to process it. You should also eat more nutritious soups such as millet soup, chicken soup, bone soup, and pork foot soup, especially the first month after giving birth.

The Chinese believe that breast-feeding should stop when the child is one or two years old. According to Chinese medical theory, when the child is older, the mother's milk's quality will become less nutritious and is not good for the child. Instead, eating food becomes more important.

From the Traditional Chinese theory, women's breast milk is from the yin blood and is produced by the spleen and stomach. Before a woman is pregnant, this body fluid exists in the form of menses. When she gets pregnant, it is restored in the Ren channel (the front middle channel) and Chong channel (relates to the productive organs) for nourishing the fetus. After giving birth, this body fluid color changes from red into white, moves upward, and becomes milk.

There are certain kinds of breast milk that show when the mother is ill and her milk is bad to the baby. Examples include milk that becomes yellow in color, is thin and clear, smells fishy, or looks like saliva. This milk is called "avoided milk" and is considered toxic in nature. Consumption of this milk can cause infantile malnutrition.

If a newborn has difficulty urinating, breast milk can be used in an herbal remedy to help this situation. The following recipe was found in the ancient book *Wai Tai*.

Cook approximately 3/4 of a cup of the mother's breast milk with 3.4 cm stalk of green onion (the white part). Bring to a boil. Divide the liquid from this process into four equal parts, and feed the baby every three hours during the day.

CAREFREE STATE

In Chinese history, there was a Confucian scholar by the name of Bo Lun who existed more than 2,000 years ago. He was well known for his love of nature and for wanting to experience as much of it as he could. He journeyed all of his life. With him, he took a servant, a shovel, and some wine in his cart. As they traveled, he told his servant that if he died along the journey to use the shovel to dig a hole and bury him. It was this carefree attitude that he carried with him that allowed him to enjoy the nature, leisure, and relaxation that he encountered along the way. This was all that mattered to him. I know that in today's world with all of our responsibilities that we cannot just pick up and leave, but we can slow down and try to be carefree even if it is for a short time.

COLDS

One of my students caught a cold when he was chopping firewood and then sat down in the shade to take a rest. He had a runny nose and headache. To help his condition, I told him to chop some fresh ginger root, put it in a cup with some dark sugar, then pour in boiling water and cover with a lid. After ten minutes, drink the hot water. This will induce sweating. He did as I requested. Later that evening he called me and happily told me that his headache and cold were gone. His cold occurred because, as he was chopping wood he was sweating and his pores were open. When he sat down to rest, he sat in the shade, which is a yin place. This allowed the wind to attack his body. To protect himself, his body closed all the pores, trapping the cold-wind and causing the cold. Ginger root is yang in nature. It has the ability to induce diaphoresis and relieve cold. Dark sugar has a warm nature as well, so it can work together with the ginger.

For colds or flu, the diet should be light, and meat should be avoided. Chapter 8 contains some recipes that may be helpful for this situation.

According to Chinese medicine there are different causes of colds, so there are different herbal formulas for different types of colds. Consulting a Chinese medical doctor will help you determine what type of herbal formula you should use. In most Chinese herbal stores there are doctors that can help you.

DRINKING WATER

I often hear people say, "Drink plenty water." How much is plenty? This is good to know because each individual's need is different. According to Chinese medicine, drinking too much water will not be beneficial to the spleen. The spleen nourishes the rest of the organs and is named the "Mother Spleen." The spleen dislikes dampness. When the spleen is healthy and strong, the qi circulation will be strong, and the body fluid circulation will be smooth.

If you are not thirsty, do not drink. When you are thirsty, do not drink a lot at a time or too fast because it will affect the qi circulation and cause illnesses such as retention of water within the body.

Drink warm water and avoid using aluminum container for water or food.

The following is an ancient true story.

Immortal Li knew an old man who was over seventy, but was as strong as a young man. He could walk on a long journey and did not feel thirsty. The old man did not have any other ways to preserve his longevity, except not drinking a lot of water as other people did. The way he practiced was that he reduced a little each day, and only drank to wet his lips when he felt thirsty.

To the Chinese, eating is a process of self-cultivation that is the message from nature. As I have mentioned earlier good dietary habits are one of the important keys to cultivation.

It is commonly believed that strong-flavored foods can harm your health without you even knowing it. Those who eat light-flavored foods will be healthier.

Most cooked, warm foods are easier to digest, especially to seniors and small children because the stomach does not have to work as hard during the digestive process as it does when raw and cold food are eaten. When a vegetable is cooked in the right way, it can be as nutritious as a raw vegetable, yet it will digest more easily.

Eat according to the season, timing, geography, your own health condition and age. Americans can enjoy foods from all over the world so try to educate yourself as to what you are putting into your body. For example, if you live in a warm or hot climate reduce the amount of meat that you consume. If you live in a damp area, you will not need as much salt as people who live in a dry area, but you may need to eat more hot peppers. Keep variety in your diet.

Before you start eating, swallow some saliva first. Do not engage in too much conversation while eating because conversation takes your mind away from the digestive process.

Chew the food until it is mushy and divide it into two to three portions to swallow. The more you chew, the more saliva you produce. Since saliva contains digestive enzymes, your food will digest more readily. Drinking hot tea after a greasy meal can aid digestion of the fat. After eating any food, rinsing your mouth with regular tea to prevent tooth decay.

Do not eat too much roasted, deep-fried food over a long period of time because fried foods can be harmful to your health.

Do not eat when you are sad, upset, or angry because the disturbed qi cannot move normally and it will disturb the digestion.

Saliva not only aids the digestion, it has other functions as well. Saliva, sweat, snivel, tears, and blood are all considered to originate from the body fluid. As a child, I often heard the adults saying that it was a bad habit to spit saliva and that people who kept spitting would have health problems. According to qigong and Chinese medical theory, if one keeps spitting saliva, his or her xin (heart-mind) will not be nourished; this can cause uneasiness.

Inability to sort out and soothe your emotions can drain your qi. I know we are human and all experience emotions, but experiencing them in excess is not good for your qi. You need to try to be in control rather that letting your emotions control you. Try to retain balance by examining your own thoughts and actions often. If you become angry, excited, or sad, for example, that is fine. Cut it short, though, and do not sink into the hole. As soon as it is over, try to forget it. In this way, you are taking care of yourself.

The following is a recipe for anxiety written by the Master Monk Shi (A.D. 617–907). This well-known recipe was carved on a rock and has been well preserved at the Hua Ting Monastery in Yunnan Province.

> *A set of good intestines with a piece of nice heart of ones own,*
> *25 grams softness, 25 grams gentleness with 1.5 grams principle.*
> *Confidence is important plus a chunk of integrity,*
> *5 grams of being a dutiful son/daughter and showing respect to the*
> *   parents,*
> *Be a complete honest person,*
> *Use both yin and yang,*
> *No limitation in convening other people.*

The way to cook the formula:

In a large-hearted pot with patience, cook slowly and with no temper, naturally with reason.

Cautions when taking the formula:

Avoid talking well but acting the opposite, benefiting oneself by harming the others, stabbing someone in the back, or hiding a dagger in a smile, or provoking troubles.

EXCESS

According to Chinese medicine and qigong theory, over-doing anything, such as too much sitting, standing, lying, or working, will not be beneficial to your health. Anything performed or experienced in excess drains energy, and excessive behaviors will not assure your happiness. Instead, they can lead to an imbalance. It is important to cultivate balance in your life and learn to know it, pass it, to share it.

Feng shui theory is an important issue in Chinese construction because it is related to the harmony of energy. The Chinese take the practice of feng shui seriously. Feng shui can be quite complex and is a science unto itself. I have translated a portion of a text from an ancient book, *Zun Sheng*, to show you just how seriously this science is taken.

The house should be built where the soil is firm and thick, brown in color and clean, and the water under the ground is deep and clean. The ceiling should be neither too high nor too low. If the ceiling is too high, the yang will be too strong, too low the yin will be too much. If the light in the house is too bright, it will effect the po (spirit that gives inspiration and courage); if too dim, it will effect the hun (soul). The windows should be closed when there is wind so that the wind will not attack the body.

Choose a location on the hill, near the water, grow plants such as bamboo, pine or cypress, and flowers that are entertaining in all the seasons.

The study room (office) should not be too big so that it will not consume the vision. The decoration can be miniature trees and rookery that both are beneficial to the health and entertaining. The best is Tian mu pine (miniature tree) from Hang Zhou City. On the wall, put up some paintings of water and mountains or classic poetry written in artistic calligraphy.

To build a pavilion in the yard, grow four cypress trees and plant a bamboo, which is used to chain the heads of the cypresses together, and weave them into a round roof.

I built a room for myself and I think it may give you some idea. It is round, a 12 square-foot room. The door faces the south. The roof is round, and its walls are squared. The room is divided into two small rooms: the front one has two windows, a sun-shape and a moon-shape, facing the east and the west. The other one opens a round window on the ceiling to receive qi from the universe.

Bamboo produces elegant air and is the symbol of noble integrity and honesty. Plant peach and willow tree in the east, the Zhe (three-bristle cudrania) and elm in the west, date and plum in the south, apricot in the north. This arrangement will bring the luck. If one grows the Chinese scholar tree in the front of the gate, his three generations will be prosperous.

It is not good to plant a tung tree (paulownia, phoenix trees) right in front of the house because it will have some negative effect to the owner.

It is not a good idea to have many ba jiao (banana) planted inside the house. There should not be a big tree in the middle of the yard, or near the house, but to have two date trees at the gate, or some willow trees is good.

The place where you often sit to rest should not have small holes in the wall because your body is unprepared, and it can be the most harmful wind. The wind goes through the hallway is also harmful especially in hot summer.

LIQUOR AND WINE

All Chinese medical books warn people that the toxin in liquor can cause "one hundred types of illnesses." Besides harming the liver and damaging the brain, drinking in excess can also cause abnormal menses, stop the production of eggs, weaken and degenerate sexual ability, and cause aging. Drinking an appropriate amount of wine, however, can be beneficial to health and can aid in the prevention of illnesses.

It is good for seniors to drink a small cup daily (about 1/3 cup) because it promotes blood and qi circulation. Some herbal wines are especially beneficial to women, such as *Ling zhi* wine, *Di huang* wine, and *Huang qi* wine; these should be taken according to direction.

Drinking warm wine is more beneficial than drinking it with ice because wine and liquor stimulate the circulation. The ice, however, disrupts this process. Do not drink tea or cold water at the same time you are drinking wine. To do so could cause illness in your lower body and lower limbs, but the symptom will not show until many years later.

MENSES AND MENOPAUSE

Menses and menopause is something that we all as women encounter during our lives. Your menses is tied to the blood. During your menses, avoid cold food and drink because they can cause blood stagnation and pain in the abdomen. According to Chinese medicine, dark pieces or clots in the blood are caused either by anger or by cold food and drink. Emotional factors strongly affect your menses, so it is important to retain a peaceful mind for a healthy menses.

Be sure during this time that you are eating nutritious foods. Avoid strong flavored, foods such as hot pepper and black and white pepper.

Avoid bathing and swimming, especially in a river or in a public swimming pool that contains chemicals. This is not good for the womb. Rest more, and avoid violent activity and heavy lifting. Choose pads that are chemical free.

If you are entering menopause, your food should be the type that can build up the liver and kidneys. Lamb cooked with black soybeans and *gui yuan* (a dried fruit that can be purchased in Chinatown), fermented soybeans cooked with lamb, and small red beans boiled are a few examples of foods that can help you. Avoid foods that are bitter or pungent in nature, hot and spicy foods, and foods that can cause dryness in the blood. Eat more food that contains fiber to avoid constipation, and do not smoke or drink liquor.

NAILS

The ancient Chinese considered it important to cut nails of both the hands and feet because they were where "the three kinds of worms hide." In modern terms, worms mean germs. Wearing fake nails is not a good idea because they can trap bacteria and fungus and cause infections. The same is true for the long nails. Many women like to polish the nails, as did the Chinese women before the early 50s in mainland China. At that time, Chinese women colored their nails by using flower juice. From my personal experience, I feel that the juice method allows the nails to breathe where acrylic polish does not.

OFFICE WORKERS

Sitting for a long time can cause qi and blood blockages in the circulation and tendon problems. You need to remind yourself to move often and do some simple exercises to promote circulation. If the air is good where you work breathe in the qigong way, stretch your shoulders and imagine that you are pulling open all of your joints. Move your waist in circles. You can also practice the Eye Exercise: look to the left and right eye corners as far as you can. Then roll your eyeballs in circles. Massage your face and head with your fingers, and knock your teeth. The important thing here is not stay stationary for long periods of time; movement does not allow the qi to stagnate.

POSITIVE ATTITUDE

The ancient teachings of the Yellow Emperor state, "It will not be effective to treat a patient that wants to die." As you try to make changes in your life or as you encounter obstacles along the way, remember to keep a positive attitude. A positive, happy-go-lucky attitude will give you positive yang energy that can help the healing process and will help you make progress in your self-cultivation.

RELAXATION

Relaxation is very important to your well-being. In this text, we have explored different qigong and meditative exercises that involve relaxing your body and mind. When I say relaxation, I do not mean recreation. I am referring instead to the resting of the mind. In the Chinese culture, a person who is not busy and who stays at home is admired as they are enjoying *qing fu*—a leisure. The Chinese believe that one can be rich, but it is difficult to buy qing fu. The well-known Grand Master Nan Huai-jin says, "Only the lucky ones can enjoy this fortune. If a qigong practitioner is able to deal with loneliness and enjoy being alone, *he or she* becomes mature." Enjoy doing nothing; enjoy relaxation and leisure time.

Because many causes of illness are due to emotional disturbances, try to be relax your mind and body if only for twenty seconds, a minute, or two during the day. It helps the body not to scatter qi and absorbs more qi from the natural world.

In April of 1996, when my dear mother came to visit us from China, we drive her around to see America. During the two-week trip, my husband was the chauffeur, and I did not practice qigong as usual. However, the warmth in my lower dan tian was more stable than anytime before. That was because with my loving, caring mother next to me, the simplicity of a child's nature was brought out. I was not taking care of the housework or working on the computer and was in the very relaxed state of qigong most of the time that she was visiting.

SENIORS

Seniors should avoid salty foods and eat less meat and more vegetables that are easier to digest. Vinegar (the dark kind made from grains is best) is good to eat for seniors because it not only prevents illness, it also softens (thins) the blood vein and reduces high blood pressure. Eat more food containing sesame seeds, but only steamed, cooked or roasted, not raw.

SEXUAL ACTIVITY

In *Tao Te Ching*, Lao Zi wrote:

> *When one's sexual desire comes naturally and the person is in a peaceful state, this person will live a long life. If one's sexual desire is from his mind, his jing will be scattered and his xin (heart-mind) will be confused, and then he will not live a long life.*

According to Chinese medical theory, sexual activity should be different according to the age and health condition of the individual. One should be aware of the changes that occur in her (or his) body. An ancient female immortal, Maiden Su, wrote:

> *When a person turns sixty, he should keep his semen and not drain it; but if he is strong and healthy, he should not force himself not to come. This is because if he forces himself not to come, it will cause illnesses.*

Some Chinese researchers also have proven that if a man restrains himself and does not come while being aroused, he could plant illness in the prostate gland.

Excessive sexual activity can drain vital energy from your kidneys. You may experience forgetfulness, soreness in your lower back, and weak knees. I have consulted two well-known Chinese qigong masters about this. One is also an M.D., and the other is a TCM doctor. They both said that before you are going to climax, hold your shen—a little bit of your awareness—at your heart. By doing so, you will keep your jing from draining. The point is sexual activity is human nature. Based on the yin-and-yang theory, only when the husband and wife enjoy themselves at the same time will making love be beneficial to the health of both.

Masturbation can cause you to lose some essence because it is not a natural release. If young people masturbate, their health will be harmed because their bodies are not mature yet. It is not a good idea to have intercourse when having your menses. According to Chinese medical thought, when a woman has menses, the inside walls of the uterus are like a fresh wound that needs to recover when the menses stops naturally. If germs are brought inside before the uterus has recovered, an infection may occur.

The following is a partial translation of a text discussing sex. As before, you can substitute the pronoun she every time he is used.

> If a man loves women with no control of himself, he will
> consume his jing*;
> If one never stops being greedy and jealous, his jing* will be scattered.
> A sage values his jing* but is generous in giving materials,
> And his bone marrow* is plenty and his bones are firm and strong....
> - Quan Yuan-qi

*Jing: the life source besides the sperm.

*Bone marrow: a concern in longevity; its condition shows if the kidneys are healthy.

In the book, *Zun Sheng*, Gao expressed himself,

> Who would not want to be with a beautiful, lovely woman? This is also the most difficult thing for a man to guard himself from over doing it (sex). Only when he learns how to preserve health and longevity, he will know that over doing (sex) will consume his kidneys, then effect his liver, and then the heart, and then the spleen, and then the lung. Then how can this person enjoy longevity? This is because a person has only limited primary qi, which cannot afford to be consumed continuously. So if his sexual desire becomes too strong, he can keep his mind on an ice mountain or something else to shift his mind and attention. Generally, he should educate himself of how to preserve health so that he will become knowledgeable. I know that discussing this subject is like talking about daily meals. It is true that who would not need to eat. But if one only eats, but does not know how to eat and when to eat, what is the value of this that he is able to eat?
>
> Do not make love when having menses; do not make love during the month after giving birth; do not make love when being in an extreme emotion (wild with joy or outrageous); and do not make love when having febrile illnesses or not having recovered from illnesses due to imbalances of yin and yang. Do not make love when the stomach is too full or is drunk, nor make love when there is thunder and storm. Do not hold the urine and make love. Do not make love when being exhausted after a long hike. Do not make love when having ulcers that are not recovered. Do not make love on the solar or lunar eclipse, nor when the temperature is extremely hot or cold.

At the health club to which I go, I saw people going into the steam room straight from the swimming pool or hot tub. This is bad for your skin because when the hot steam opens up the pores, the skin will absorb chemicals in the pool.

If your skin is dry, try placing a few drops of olive oil into your bath water to help condition your skin. Try to use soaps that contain ginseng or flower pollen; they are also condition the skin.

When you apply lotion to your face, apply it from the cheeks up to the forehead, massage and press the acupoints around the eyes, press the eyelids gently on the eyeballs.

Eating right and practicing qigong is the best way to improve the skin and prevent wrinkles. Rub your hands together until they are hot; then dry-wash your face, neck, head with your hands as many times as you can. If you wear make-up, you can do this before going to bed and when you get up.

Many foods and herbs can benefit the skin such as Yin er soup (silver mushroom), Chinese date soup, Yi yi ren grains, and tomatoes.

SLEEPING

To the Chinese, it is just as important to keep your body in a harmonious state when you are asleep as while you are awake. Try using a pillow that is adjustable and supportive. The most common, inexpensive, and supportive pillows in China are made of buckwheat shells. They are good to use in hot and cold seasons. You can also find pillows with herbal fillings for special purposes. The bed should be high above the ground to avoid the yin qi from the ground. Quality of sleep, not quantity, is more important. According to qigong and Chinese medical theory, at night between 7–11:00 P.M., more yin qi is produced. When a person is sleeping during these hours, the qi stays in the joints. During the hours of 12–2:00 A.M., the yang qi is produced; if you sleep on your side with the top leg slightly curled on the bottom leg, the body fluid will promote qi and blood to circulate better and to move to the lower dan tian. The ancient Chinese described that sleeping with the body curled like a deer could store the qi and make it easier for the qi to move into the lower dan tian. When you don't have much time to relax in your bed in the morning, before you get up, you may simply turn on your back first to stretch your limbs. Stretch your arms up above your head and pull your legs downward, stretching all your joints . Then you turn on your right side and curl your body like a deer for a minute to allow the qi to return to the lower dan tian and then get up. Doing this puts your mind and body in harmony before beginning the day.

The ancient book, *Zun Sheng*, says,

Before you sleep, do not think of bad things but nice things, think of a good deed that you did. It helps prevent bad dreams. If someone often has nightmare, get 15 grams of Zhu sha (cinnabar) and put it in a small red bag (cotton or silk), and put the bag on the head inside the hat when you are going to sleep. When sleeping, do not put the feet high. Do not put your hands on the chest or you will have you have dreams.

When you feel hot, do not go back to sleep right after drinking water. Do not talk in bed when you are going to sleep. Do not tell others about your dreams.

If you have fears before you go to bed, visualize the sun or the moon inside your chest or on your forehead. If you go to urinate, it is good to keep your eyes open.

It is better to keep your mouth shut when sleeping so that the good qi will not be drained.

The Chinese *Materia Medica* says,

Do not use a light to wake a sleeping person so that his shen will not be disturbed. If someone suddenly loses consciousness, do not turn a light on his face at once; instead, use the fingernail to press his Ren zhong point (the hallow part under the nose) or bite the nail of his thumb and spit on his face.

Do not sleep on your back if there is thunder.

The following ancient advice is still popular and is good for seniors, too.

When you wake up, exhale twice to release the dirty qi from the night, then rub the palms until hot, massage the sides of nose, then the eyes and eye brows. Then pull your ears up and down, forth and back, each five to seven times. Then your hands hold the head, use index and the middle fingers to knock the back of the head, 24 times. Then you stretch your body, exercise your two arms as if you were shooting an arrow to the left and then right, each five to seven times. Then you stretch the two legs and hold them back, five to seven times. Next, you knock your teeth and rinse your mouth with saliva, swallow 3 times. After these exercises, you rest for a minute, and get up and drink a little warm water, three to five swallows. It is good to have some soft rice soup eaten with cooked vegetable in the morning. Then massage the abdomen and take a short walk.

To massage the abdomen, make clockwise circles: start from the navel, move gradually up touching the rib-chest and down to the top of pubic bones; then make circles counterclockwise, gradually smaller, and back to the navel. Pause for a minute.

STERILITY

For those women who were born healthy but cannot conceive a child, Chinese medicine looks at three main causes. This problem can be quite complex, however; so many times there are many other contributing factors other than the major three. Such problems are related to kidney deficiency. Kidneys produce jing that is directly related to the reproduction system. Kidney (water element) is the mother of the liver (wood element). Stagnation of the liver-qi will stop jing from moving and prevent conception from occurring. The best option for a woman who has fertility problems is to go to see a Chinese medical doctor and get examined. Because this area is very complicated, the doctor can best decided what the problem is.

Women who have such problems should avoid smoking and liquor, which will cause harm to the egg. They should also avoid pungent foods such as black pepper and hot pepper, because they stimulate the liver. Roasted or fattening food should also be avoided so that the stagnation will not get worse.

SWEATING

When you are sweating, it is a good idea to avoid wind because it may cause wind syndrome such as such as swelling migratory pain in joints, colds, or arthritis-like symptoms. According to Chinese medical theory, sweat is related to the different organs. Sweat that results from eating hot food is related to the stomach; sweat that results from being scared is related to the heart; sweat that results from a long hike is related to the kidneys; sweat due to being frightened when running is related to the liver; and sweat caused by hard, physical work is related to the spleen. It is also believed that if sweat drops on the food, the food becomes inedible.

TEETH

It is good to exercise your jaws and gums to promote healthy teeth. Chew some chewy food, not just soft and easy-to-chew foods. This way, your teeth will get exercise and become firmer. Some old Chinese like to chew dried chestnuts for strong teeth. The ancient Chinese considered it more important to brush the teeth before going to bed than in the morning because the food remaining between the teeth after eating will produce harmful germs and harm the teeth and gums.

THIN WOMEN

Thin women need to consume sweet and moist foods, should avoid hot and black pepper, and should not eat a lot of lamb. According to Chinese medicine, being thin is a kind of blood deficiency, usually too much internal heat.

WALKING

Always remember the qigong way of walking is relaxed, not fast. When the air is fresh, you can inhale and exhale deeply in rhythm, all way to and from the lower dan tian. Before finishing the walk, swallow some saliva to gather qi into your lower dan tian.

WEIGHT CONTROL

According to Chinese medicine, if you are overweight usually much phlegm has been produced inside the system and dampness has accumulated in the spleen. With this in mind, you should eat more foods that benefit the spleen and release dampness and that are easy to digest. Because each individual is different, you should be diagnosed by an experienced Chinese medical doctor.

Eating right plus getting the appropriate amount of exercise is the key for losing weight and for staying in shape. Never skip your breakfast and lunch for eating a big dinner. To the Chinese lunch is much more important than dinner; eating a light dinner is a wise way to live.

In this chapter I have covered a wide variety of subjects and have presented you with a Chinese point of view on them. I hope that by doing so that I may have opened the door to some understanding to the Chinese culture and how the principles that we have discussed so far in the text of this book help to contribute to those opinions.

Prevention is the essential issue, and you will find this in the following translations from ancient Chinese texts that I have provided for you. Such texts have been valuable resources to the Chinese people for thousands of years. As a child, I was given the following advice by adults; now I found them in an ancient text,

> Do not bathe when you are hungry; do not shower when you are full or have eye illness; do not wash your head with cold water which may cause the head wind; do not wash your head when you are sweating; do not go to bed with wet hair. Do not sit on a stone that is heated by the sun, which may cause piles; do not sit on a cold stone which may cause hernia. Do not sleep on your stomach. If the weather is too hot and it effects your skin, do not wash your face until the skin's temperature becomes normal.

Although in the following poem "he" is the major character, "she" can also share the wisdom.

TRANSLATIONS

"Ten Ways of Prolonging Life"
— Gao Lian

Yin (female) and yang (male) make love harmoniously, touch in proper and coordinating ways; this prolongs life.

The couple who masters the right methods and enjoys inside the room, but forget it when going out; this benefits their longevity.

He does not masturbate, nor does he love young boys, his life can be lengthened.

If he keeps away from heavily made-up women and prostitutes, his life will be prolonged.

When he values his jing as gold and his body as treasure, his life is prolonged.

When he learns to take tonic herbal formulas to build up his lower primary*, it prolongs his life.

When one is not infatuated with other women and his mind is not lost, he has prolonged his life.

When one does not have vain hopes and does not have sex in his dreams, it prolongs his life.

When being young, he is not reluctant to sexual activity, when being old, he knows when to stop; this will allow him to enjoy longevity.

If one can avoid a beauty as avoiding a tiger, and not lose control in sexual activity; he will enjoy longevity.

*Primary: the life source at the lower dan tian

The following poems were written by Immortal Sun, Si-miao (A.D. 581–722), who was a well-known Taoist physician and who is called the King of Medicine. If you follow his advice, you should be healthy in all the seasons.

First poem:

"Poetry of Preserving Health"

Between the Heaven and the earth, human beings are the most precious,
Your head is the symbol of the Heaven, your feet are the symbol of the earth.
Learn to take good care of the body given by your parents,
Then you can enjoy the five "happiness": longevity, health and peace, wealth, moral integrity, and a good ending (of which longevity is the most important).

The "three avoids" must be known in personal hygiene:
Outrages, extreme anxieties (over sex), and excessive drinking (wine and liquor).
If one of the three is involved,
You must be alert to harming and draining the primary qi (life force).

To seek longevity, be on guard against your temper,
Without producing the fire of longings, your xin (mind/heart) will retain peace,
Then the wood (liver) would not be burned into ashes but live,
And your life will be prolonged as you have guarded against the temper.

Greediness can be never satisfied, which only causes the essence inside to be forgotten,
To nudge your brain in continuously thinking will consume your primary shen,
Which eventually can consume your body completely and drain your qi,
What then is there left to protect your health?

When too much of the mind is taxed, consumption is caused,
When too much of the body is weakened, fatigue happens,
When too much of the shen is harmed, xu (deficiency) is caused,
When the qi is exhaust, life stops.

To learn to preserve health,
Retain an unperturbed, happy mind and seldom get angry,
Be honest and decent, worries will be removed,
Cultivate yourself good principles to avoid vexation.

In spring, you exhale xu- to soothe the liver and improve the vision,
In summer exhale (k)her- to soothe your xin (heart-mind),
In autumn you exhale Ss- to soothe the lung,
In winter you exhale chui- to soothe the kidneys.
Hu- exhalation is good to do in all the seasons to soothe your spleen
    and aid to digestion,
To release heat inside, you can exhale the sound of xi-.

It is good to comb your hair often and exercise the qi,
Knock often your teeth and swallow your saliva,
To retain longevity do the Head Exercise
And massage your face often.

Eat some sweet but not too much sour in spring,
Eat some pungent but not much salty in winter,
Eat more pungent but less bitter natured in summer,
Eat some sour food but reduce bitter natured in autumn.
Avoid too salty and not much sweet in all the seasons,
Then your five organs will be safe naturally.
To make the food tasty is easy but not to avoid getting sick,
So to reduce all the flavors is for staying healthy.*

In chilly spring do not wear thin clothes,
In hot summer change clothes when getting sweaty,
In autumn and winter, adjust the coldness and add clothes gradually,
And do not wait until sick then have to take medicine.

Hot summer is the season that is most difficult to maintain health,
Avoid drinking much ice water because of the latent yin inside,
Avoid eating too much cold-nature fruit like melons and peaches and
    raw food,
Which are the prevention from getting pathogenic type of dysentery in
    autumn and winter.

If physically strong but with weak kidneys, one better
    avoid sex for a time,
But to nourish the kidneys,
And reinforce the jing (life source) and moderate sex,
Avoid fattening foods and deficiency in order to build up your kidneys.

Too full a stomach can harm your shen (heart-spirit), too hungry can
    harm the stomach,
Being too thirsty can harm the blood, but drinking too much can harm
    the qi.
Do not eat much when hungry, do not drink much when thirsty,

This will prevent from getting a large abdomen, and not harm the
heart and lung.

Stop drinking before drunk, stop eating when not feeling hungry,
So sickness will not happen.
Humans depend on eating right to preserve health,
Avoid extremes then life will become comfortable and easy.

After a meal, take a short relaxed walk,
And massages the abdomen gently to aid digestion.
At night massages your gum and teeth (with tongue) to get more saliva
and swallow,
And remember to exhale the (k)her- to release dirty qi from the lower
abdomen.

Drinking moderate amount of wine can mold temperament,
But drinking much can lead one hundred kinds of illnesses.
When the lung is injured the body will be harmed as a damaged
canopy of the carriage,
Severe coughing will consume the shen (heart-spirit) and eventually
cause death.

Be careful not to salt in the drinking tea,
Which will be like to invite a thief into your house.
When the lower limbs feel cold, it will lead to emaciation,
Which has shown your kidneys and spleen have become weakened, and
be cautious not to become sicker.

When sleeping or sitting, do not let the cold wind attack your head and
back,
If the head is attacked by cold wind, his life will be shortened.
It is bad to sleep in the wind when the stomach is full or drunk,
Because the wind can attack the five organs to cause calamities and
diseases.

Wild geese have their principle, dogs have their ties of friendship,
Even the black corps have their etiquette and must face north.
When a person with no ethics and unscrupulous behavior eats such
animals,
Neither the Heaven, earth, immortals, nor the ghosts will be pleased.

To preserve health, moderate the five flavors,
Lack of moderation will only cause harm.
Do not ever cause yang deficiency that can cause the jing to exhaust,
Which will cause his face to look haggard and various kinds of illnesses
to occur.

No matter if at home or on a trip,
When there are thunders and lightening,
It is better to sit quietly and be cautious,
Quietly check your thoughts and respect the nature.

If deeply involved in conjugal, exceedingly sentimental love, he will lose
    the freedom,
If indulges in fame and gains, will there be an end to life to be bogged
    down?
By relaxing and letting go, he will keep the remaining luck in his life,
Then he can avoid premature aging.

It is not easy to create this world,
How can one not feel gratitude to having plenty of food and warm
    clothes?
To appreciate the bounties bestowed by the universe,
Burn incense to be thankful.

What will he or she think when enjoying health and longevity?
His or her xin (mind/heart) should retain ease, and do more benevo-
    lent deeds,
And treasure their lives, bodies, and qi.
Gentlemen and ladies with moral integrity,
Please memorize my 'Poem for Preserving Health.'

* Five flavors: They are: sour, salty, sweet, pungent, bitter, each
related to one of the five organs. Bitter attributes to the heart,
pungent to the lungs, sour to the liver, sweet to the spleen, salty
to the kidneys.

Second poem:

Extreme anger hurts the qi,
The train of thoughts consumes the shen.
When the shen becomes tired, then the heart is overworked.
Then the qi becomes deficient, which leads a person to get sick easily,
This is why one should avoid extreme joy or sadness.
He should always eat appropriate meals,
And avoid getting drunk at night,
Nor get angry in the morning.
When going to bed, he knocks his teeth 36 times,
Before getting up in the morning,
He rinses his mouth with the saliva and swallows.
So the evil factors and spirits will not harm him easily
Because he has gotten plenty jing and qi.

Prevention relates to the five organs,
So one should avoid being excessive of the flavors.
His temper has been exercised gentle resulted to have preserved his qi,
And peaceful and happy will be what his mind and heart retain to be.

Chapter 7

*To be angry in Chinese is called
"sheng qi"—to create qi.*

Qi, Food, and Herbs

PRINCIPLES

In this chapter, I will cover the basics of how foods and herbs are integrated into the cultivation process. Such principles come from the roots of ancient China. They are best explained in the *Nei Jing*. I have translated the following passage so that it may help you understand.

> *Yin and yang is the Tao of the universe which is in constant change. After you have learned the principle of yin and yang, you will be like a child who is always with your parents being protected. This is because you will become perceptive of the causes as well as the truth. The changing of the four seasons is for the growing and restoring of living things. Wise people will adapt into the changes to protect themselves, and learn the way to keep good health. Ignorant people will act in diametrically opposite ways with the changes and harm themselves.*

The yin and yang principle is the philosophy of prevention: the balancing of yin and yang in all aspects of your life to suit constant changes. All Chinese herbal formulas and food recipes for prevention and treatment were designed based on this principle. Holistic medicine looks at the whole picture of a situation before it puts an herb or food to use, including the nature of the herb, its good side, its harmful side, and which ones can or cannot be used together to increase or decrease the healing effect.

Certain herbs and foods benefit men more than women or vice versa. The foods and herbs used in treatment are designed to accommodate the differences between each individual. Throughout history, much experimental data was compiled that perfected this science.

Western medicine often targets treatment of the symptom of an illness. The eastern way is to treat the root cause of the illness rather than focus on the symptoms at hand. I know these ideas may seem quite foreign to you but, with a little bit of guidance, this knowledge can help you to get your body into a more harmonious state.

In eastern philosophy, many times the answer to a question is very different from the western way of looking at things. If something works, that is a good enough reason to use it; things do not always have to be proved in a laboratory setting. For example, an autopsy allows a doctor to look inside a corpse and see physically the organs and maybe even see the cause of the death, yet he or she cannot look inside a living person and see the qi that is keeping the patient alive. Like the qi, many different aspects of the Chinese culture have no modern research as to why and how they function; a good example is sesame seeds. Chinese consider black sesame seeds to be good for preserving longevity, and they never eat raw sesame seeds. The Chinese do not eat raw sesame seeds because the ancient teaching says that eating raw sesame seeds causes hair loss. Do I have a scientific reason for this? I do not. I only know it is based on the thousands years of research and experiments.

From eastern and western viewpoints the concept of diet and nutrition have different meanings. The concept of nutrition in Western medicine looks to the elements that are found in food and how they effect the body. To the Chinese it is defined in qi. Grand qigong master Ming-tang Xu writes, "Nutriology is different from diet for healing. Chinese diet is to bring the body back to balance. Still, back to balance does not mean back to origin (spiritual purpose)."

Because of these fundamental differences, illness and its treatment is looked at differently. For example, if a person angers easily and is easily irritated, traditional Chinese medicine would say that perhaps the liver qi has stagnated; therefore, the liver would be treated, and the anger would subside. One time I heard a man consulting a radio doctor about controlling his anger. This man was in tears when he was asking for help. The only advice he received was to watch his manner and behavior and to be nice to his family. The physical reasons for his anger were not addressed at all. Perhaps if this man was advised as to proper herbal formulas and diet and maybe some acupuncture treatments, then the toxin that caused his anger would be released.

The Chinese put great emphasis on using diet and herbs to prevent illness before it begins. This is a philosophy that is integrated into the culture from ancient times. The Yellow Emperor said, "To eat and exercise to prevent is more important than to heal. A good physician will treat an illness before it happens." This means that as we are part of nature, we have to eat right to stay healthy, to heal, and to follow the constant changes in our body as well as in the natural world.

You may wonder how one begins to understand the diagnostic process. I can tell you that it takes years of experience and study to be able to do it. However, I can provide you with a brief explanation that will at least give you an idea of what is involved. The Five Element Theory found in Chapter 2 is one of the applications that Chinese physicians use in the prevention of illness and the promotion of longevity. To do so, you have to learn how our organs are related to one another based on the elements and how these elements interact with the qi that flows in our body. In addition you also need to understand how our bodies relate to nature. The interactions of the five elements also express a theory of the mutual promotion and restraint between the foods we eat, the herbs we take, and their effect on our organs. As you can see, these theories get quite complicated and need a much deeper explanation that I can cover in this text. My purpose here is to give you an idea why diet is so important to cultivation and to provide you with some common Chinese remedies for common ailments.

Understanding diet and the Five Element Theory gives you insight to understand why certain areas of the body or certain organs were being treated. For example, you would know that for soothing your liver that is disturbed by anger, you can take herbal formulas such as Shu gan wan or Jia wei xiao yao wan, depending on your liver's needs. You would also know to pay attention to the organs that are directly related to the liver. You would see if your heart-fire is burning, which would harm your liver; you would check if your kidney-water is nourishing your liver-wood. You would also check if there is anything wrong in your spleen and stomach—the earth center because all the other four organs are affected by the center.

When you visit traditional Chinese medical doctors, they are concerned with the activity of your qi. They check it by feeling your pulse, checking the color of your face, examining your palms, checking the coating on your tongue, checking your breath, and your feces. Because each of these conditions is unique to the individual, it is the individual that decides the diet and herbal formulas that she or he receives. The differences between individuals such as age, sex, health condition, lifestyle, and emotions are taken into consideration as well.

FOODS AND QI

Chinese people eat balanced meals according to the season, as well as according to individual needs. Although diagnosis of illness can be complicated, eating to promote balance can be quite understandable. If Chinese people who do not have a college education or even a high school diploma have learned how to eat to adapt to the changes, so will you. As long as you do not blindly follow others but instead eat to feel, you will become your own expert. The key here is self-education. The following are some examples of how food is used in healthcare—treatment and prevention.

By Season

A great example of seasonal eating is not eating too much ginger root in autumn. In the fall season, people do not eat too much ginger root because it is against nature. Autumn is the season for all living things to store qi but ginger root's function is to disperse qi; this is opposite of what is supposed to be happening during the autumn season. You should eat food that is not dispersing and foods like radish that prevent diseases that are usually caused in cold weather. Cooked radish cleanses phlegm that is often caused by cold temperature. Eating raw radish promotes qi circulation and cleanses heat. This is an example of how diet is important according to season.

By Geography

The following is an example of to how to eat according to geographic location. If you live in a humid, hot area, you should eat more rice than wheat and less meat; meat and wheat produce much more heat than rice, but this climate provides more than enough heat to your body. Rice is also easier to digest and will not make your spleen and stomach do extra work. Your spleen especially has to work on the dampness in this humid, hot condition because the spleen does not like dampness (according to the Five Element Theory). If you live in a cold, dry area, you should eat more wheat and butter; they produce more heat to promote the circulation of qi. When the body is too cold, the qi circulation inside the body shrinks. According to Chinese theory, this is why you curl your body up when you feel cold. You can eat some meat if you like. However, be cautious about meat. Meat is a more complicated subject that I will not discuss much in this book. You will find a lot information about meat in my upcoming *Herbal Food* book.

HOW CAN WE BRING QI INSIDE OUR BODIES INTO BALANCE AND HARMONIZE OUR QI BY EATING?

I would like to begin this subject with a Chinese story. This story dates back to the Shang Dynasty (c. 16th-11th century B.C.). The Prime Minister, Yin Yi, was a gourmet cook and dietary expert. His specialty was using spices. He thought that if the spices were used in a balanced and harmonious way, the dishes would be both tasty and beneficial to health and that, otherwise, they could be harmful. He used this philosophy to carry over to his method of political ruling as well. He developed China into a peaceful, strong nation by creating the foundation of the Shang Dynasty that lasted several hundred years. His cooking philosophy and experiences still play an important role in Chinese cooking even today.

Yin Yi's theory was based on the Yellow Emperor's philosophy that originated from Taoism. This theory addresses how to get the energy—qi—from food to balance the yin and yang energy in the body and to adapt in the natural world. According to Chinese culture, all foods have their own nature. Foods that belong to the same nature possess slightly different degrees of yin (coolness) and yang (warmth) and can function in slightly different manners. Examples include black, brown, and white sugar; various peppers; wheat grown in cold climates verses wheat grown in warm climates. According to "Ben Tsao," "Wheat grown in a cold climate 'contains the four seasons qi,' which is better than wheat grown in a warm climate." A food's nature and qi can also change due to the way you cook it. For example, roasted and deep-fried food contains more heat-fire qi. Steamed and boiled foods contain gentle qi. Because of our bodies' natural changes, the same food can be beneficial to a fifty year-old person, but may not be good to an elderly person even if they have the same illness.

Nature and Flavor

So far, I have mentioned that during different times of the day our organs become more active and that different sounds and emotions can do the same. This is true with various foods and flavors as well. If you can learn to adapt to the natural cycle and eat according to the needs of your body, then you can balance the qi and put yourself in a more harmonious state. In the Yellow Emperor's *Nei Jing*, it says, "To eat can produce qi and benefit jing, nourish qi and protect the health. But one can also eat to harm himself."

According to diet in western terms, as I understand it, foods get classified according to nutritional information. Foods become measurements of the amounts of fat, protein, and carbohydrates that they contain, and people eat them according to these measurements. Little is placed on any effect the food may have except for its impact on weight control. As foods are transported worldwide with ease it is very easy to obtain foods that are out of season. Eating in this manner will easily put you in a state of imbalance. A Chinese diet will take into consideration many different factors to help you achieve a more balanced state. The Chinese diet classifies food according to its nature. These natures are defined in terms of five flavors: sweet, sour, bitter, salty, and pungent. Be careful so as not to misinterpret the concept of flavor. The five flavors refer to the nature of the foods as well as the taste. Sweet foods would include foods that are sugars, sugary fruits, and chestnuts. Sour foods would be lemon, limes, plums or those foods that possess a sour nature. Pungent foods are types such as black and hot pepper. Bitter-natured foods are not just bitter like bitter melon, but those that function in discharging such as honey and watermelon. Salty foods include salt and those foods that have a high salt content such as seaweed. The foods' natures are important because they affect you internally. The Chinese have studied for thousands of years the cause and effect of the natures of foods. In the ancient

Chinese writing, the Yellow Emperor's *Nei Jing*, such causes and effects are discussed. The text states that the liver is affected by sour; the heart is affected by bitter, the spleen by sweet, the kidneys by salt, and the lungs by pungent. The following is a translation directly from the text. Keep in mind as you will read that, just like the concept of qi has been ingrained in the Chinese culture, these ideas are second nature to the Chinese.

> *The universe feeds people with the five qi, the earth feeds people with the five flavors. People eat the five flavored foods and store them in the stomach and intestines to nourish the five qi. When the qi is in harmony, it produces life, body fluid, and shen (spirit) is born. When eating the foods that their flavors and qi are in harmony, they regulate the circulation to benefit the jing (essence) and qi (vital energy).*

It is important to eat a wide variety of foods and not the same thing all of the time. Each of the five flavors can also bring about a bodily response. For example, sweet can slow down symptoms of illness, sour can obstruct movements, bitter can reduce heat and moisture, salty can soften hardness, and pungent can promote energy circulation. Now you can see that an understanding of how the different natures and flavors of foods you consume can affect your organs. You can use this knowledge, the yin and yang theory, and a little thought to help yourself. For example, if you have a fever it means that you have an excess of internal heat; you can use foods that are bitter to break the fever because bitter foods reduce heat. The approach to eating well is one that uses a lot of common sense; you just need an introduction to the rules.

Sensations

There are a few other basic concepts of Chinese diet to which I would like to introduce you. In addition to the natures and flavors, we need to look at the sensations that foods produce in your body in relation to hot and cold. There are five sensations; they are hot, cold, warm, cool, and neutral. It is equally important that you become familiar with which foods produce which sensations. For example, if you are overheated during the summer, eat a food that will get rid of the internal heat, one that produces a cooling sensation—watermelon or mung bean soup.

Constitution

The last basic concept states that you need to apply these ideas to the constitution of your body at the time. There are six constitutions that I will speak of in terms of health conditions. They are hot and cold, dry and damp, excessive and deficient. When creating a balanced diet for yourself, it is important to understand your constitution because it is unique to you. This will cause a diet to vary greatly from person to person. I will explain these constitutions to you generally so that you get the idea of how this works.

❖ Hot and cold. If you are a hot individual, you tend to be hot and thirsty and prefer cold drinks often; your tongue can appear red, you urinate infrequently, and you can have hard stools. If you are cold, you tend to feel cold, you prefer hot or warm drinks, your complexion tends to be pale, your tongue can appear light in color or whitish, your urine will be clear, and your stool will be loose.

❖ Dry and damp. If you are dry, you may have a dry cough and dry skin; you may have trouble gaining weight and may often suffer from constipation. If you are damp, you may easily gain weight from water retention, your tongue may appear glossy, and you may often feel tired and sluggish.

❖ Deficient and excessive. If you possess a deficient condition, your energy will be low, and you will feel weak a lot of the time. You may experience heart palpitations as well as shortness of breath. Your tongue may appear without coating, and you will tend to be underweight. If you are excessive you tend to have an abundance of energy and you tend to have a reddish complexion and can suffer from hypertension or heart disease.

Therefore, to eat a balanced diet you need to be able to recognize you constitution and basically eat foods and herbs advised by a Chinese medical doctor that will produce the opposite effect. For example, based on what we have discussed so far, if you determine that your constitution is hot then you need to eat more foods that produce a cooling effect or that possess cold energy—this means the nature of food, not necessarily cold food and drink. You would also need to consider eating the flavor bitter because bitter will dispel heat. Eating in this manner will help you to balance your body's qi.

HERBS

When you are dealing with herbs, it is important to obtain as much information about them as possible. I have seen cases especially with popular herbs where the information about them is incomplete. This can be a dangerous situation. I have also seen exaggerated claims about herbs as well. I once saw a letter from a medical practitioner with this mandate: "Take your herb books and throw them in the trash!" This doctor announced that only his "miracle ten herbs" have the "cures of many diseases." I read the letter and was shocked by how ignorant this doctor was. Maybe he has helped some patients. However, how can ten herbs replace this colorful world in which a human being's body is the most complicated? It needs variety, no matter how small amount that element is.

I have mentioned this before, but I will say it again because it is so important: Educate yourself as much as you can. This knowledge can be incorporated into cultivation. Remember cultivation incorporates not only the practice of qigong but the integration of balanced eating habits and some degree of Chinese herbal medicine. The more educated you are, the more you can cultivate. In the Yellow Emperor's *Nei Jing*, it says,

> It is wrong to say that chronic illness cannot be healed. A good doctor is an expert in using his needles to treat the disease like pulling out a thorn from the skin; or to washing off dirty things from the body; or as to untying a rope knot, to unblock the silted up qi channels. A good doctor will prescribe according to the qi changing in the seasons, the changes of the weather, the geography, and the individual.

HERBAL FORMULAS FOR WOMEN

Some herbal formulas are designed differently to accommodate the biological differences between men and women. There have been outstanding Chinese medical books written only for women such as *The Complete Effective Prescription for Women's Diseases* written by a qigong master-physician, Chen Zi-ming (A.D. 1190–1272), and *Gynecology and Obstetrics* written by Fu Qing-zhu (A.D. 1644). *The Complete Effective Prescription for Women's Diseases* is the most complete monograph on gynecology and obstetrics in the world, while *Gynecology and Obstetrics* includes many poems used for diagnosis, treatments, and diet recipes. Many Chinese medical books supply plenty of herbal formulas and diet recipes for diseases that afflict women. They often focus on first building up the blood based on the age of the patient. For example, before a girl has menses and after her menopause is over, the food recipes and qigong practice do not differ that much because they do not possess their menses—so that is not a concern. When a girl has menses, however, her food should have some differences. She should avoid pungent types of foods because they speed up blood flow. During her menses and right after giving birth, she should eat more food that builds up her spleen-stomach so as to ensure the building up of her blood. Some recipes for such cases are included in Chapter 8. It is also believed that a woman who has her menses should not do heavy lifting or work in cold water. In China when a woman gives birth, her vacation time from her job is fifty-six days. This is in accordance with the life cycle of the fetus, which changes every seven days. Basically, it will take almost this length of time for the woman who gave birth to recover.

UNDERSTAND THE HERBS YOU ARE TAKING

I have noticed with western medicine that a prescription drug can be given to a vast number of people (as long as they are not allergic) that possess similar symptoms. This is not true with herb use. Because everyone is different, the types of herbs they might use for similar symptoms may differ. There are, however, some cases where I have seen misinformation about herbs that may cause you to think that they can be used in a generic sense. One example is *Dang gui*. The word, *Dang*, means it is time and *gui* means to return. Dang gui has the function to bring blood back or to return blood back. I recently saw on TV a doctor who was discussing the harm of over-dosing drugs. He has helped his patients overcome these effects by using herbal medicine. He was promoting the use of Dang gui, yet he was using it very much the same way you might take a prescription medication. A Chinese medical doctor will not promote one single herb to all users. Most herbs' side effects are mellow and gentle, but still, they are used with other herbs to bring out their best function and to fit the individual. Dang gui is a great herb for treating illnesses related to blood problems, especially for women. But according to Chinese medicine, there are different types of blood deficiencies. When you order Dang gui from a Chinese herbal company, you will have to tell them what you are using it for because as many other herbs, the different parts of this root function in different ways. For example, the head of the root stops bleeding; the root body harmonizes the blood, and its tail removes blood stasis. The ancient Chinese doctors warned people that if one did not know how to use the root, they should not use it at all. Aside from using the different parts of the root it can also be processed differently according to the condition you are treating as well. For example, in most cases, Dang gui can be processed in wine, but not for the patient having a complication of phlegm. In this case, Dang gui should be processed with ginger. If the patient has a headache, Dang gui root should be cooked in wine, and this patient should only take the surface part of the wine. If the patient also has chest pain, then grind Dang gui into powder and mix the powder in wine and take it. If there is blood in the patient's urine, cook the root in wine and have the patient drink it. If the patient has heat in the blood, it will be used with *Sheng di huang* and *Tiao qin*. If there is only a blood deficiency, assist it with Ginseng and *Shi zhi*. For the same illness, the recipe for a virgin will be different from that for a married woman.

Additionally, Dang gui's nature is also affected by geography. To remove blood stasis, the kind grown in Sichuan is more powerful for nourishing the blood; Dang gui from middle China is gentler. Dang gui should not be used together with Lu ru, wet wheat flour, Chang pu, Hai zao (seaweed), or raw ginger root.

Now you see, using herbs is not that simple. Chinese diet and herbal medicine work in totally different ways than western medicine, and it is very important to know as much as you can about an herb before you reach for a bottle in a health food store. Before you choose an herbal product, please make sure that the information that you obtain about the herb is from a trained professional such as a Chinese medical doctor.

I hope that I have at least provided you with a basic understanding of these sciences so that you can see how, in the process of cultivating qi, it is not only important to meditate and practice qigong but also to include balanced eating habits using well chosen food and herbs. I will provide you with a list of foods and herbal remedies that are commonly used in China as a reference for your cultivation process. Remember as I have said before, this book is designed to introduce you to the idea of what qigong and cultivation is and how you may incorporate it into your life. It is important that you continue to educate yourself on these subjects. What I have provided for you here are basic concepts that may provide you with a foundation on which to build.

I would like to conclude this chapter with the following ancient wisdom:

"The Ways that Prolong Life"

— Gao Lian

*The following will affect eighty percent if one learns what to avoid when
  eating and drinking:*

Cooked vegetables and rice soup can be eaten plenty with pleasure,

Eat without extravagant wishes but enjoy what you have,

When you do not like to kill to satisfy your taste buds,

And cannot harden your heart to see an animal to be cooked alive,

You understand the pain of a crying animal when being killed.

You do not seek delicious meat of an animal from far away,

*Nor do you eat a farming ox or cow and animals that have moral
  integrity.*

You do not eat raw fish or sleep right after eating meat,

Nor do you drink much wine to confuse your own nature.

You do not like to chop meat to cook,

*Nor do you indulge in strong tastes that poison your five organs'
  sensors.*

You do not eat left over food touched by birds or mice,

Nor do you eat the animal meat from a hunter, or lay a trap for food,

Or the eat the meat of the animal that was raised by yourself.

Do not punish the servants if the food is not cooked right,

And think of each meal precious and know where it comes from,

So you will not waste any grain.

Do not eat when you are not hungry so to avoid harming the spleen,

Do not drink fast when you are thirsty.

Nor do you eat much at once when you are starving,

Do not leave on an empty stomach in the morning,

And never eat until you feel full in the evening.

A wise Emperor Qian Long lived eighty-eight years of healthy
life. His experience is in the following poems.

"The 'Ten Often'"

Knocking the teeth, swallow your saliva often,

Beating the head back with the fingers to improve your hearing,

Rubbing the nose sides hot often,

Turning the eyeballs far and round,

Everyday your hands massage your feet and face,

And your palms massage your abdomen in circles,

Remember to stretch your four limbs,

And do not forget to contract your anus gently and often."

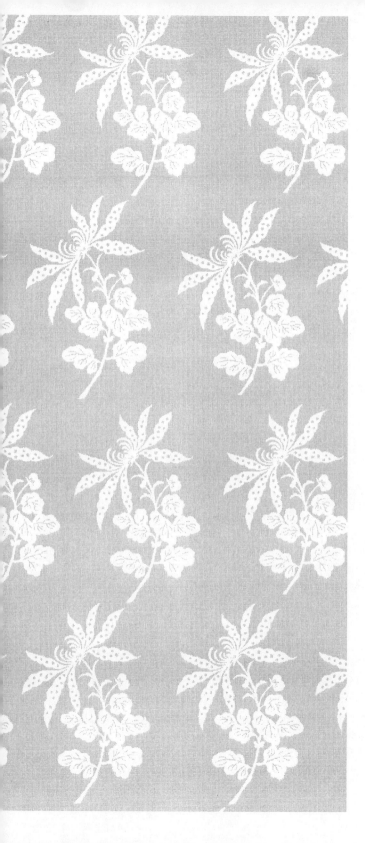

Chapter 8

"The Four Not"
  Do not talk while eating,
  Do not have conversation in bed
  before sleeping,
  Do not drink until drunk,
  Do not be obsessive with beautiful
  men/women.

To mean a senior in good health,
Chinese say, "Her/his jing qi shen
look good."

Herbal Remedies

Food and herbal remedies aim to put the whole body, not just a specific part of it, in harmony. In Chapter 7, I touched on the basics of Chinese herbology and food practice. Chinese herbology is, however, quite complex and requires years of study to become knowledgeable in the subject. If you wish to treat yourself or your family in the herbal way I suggest that you consult an herbal physician who can guide you in the process.

In 1959, some Chinese researchers collected from different ancient Chinese medical books information about a total of 152 kinds of foods and herbs that have been used since ancient times for the prevention of aging. Their recipes are designed for healthy people, for different ages, for different health problems, and for different seasons. Therefore, a large quantity of food and herbal remedies are still commonly practiced within the Chinese culture.

In the text that follows I will explain how one would go about preparing herbal wines, teas, soups, candies, snacks, and infusions. I have also translated some of the commonly used ancient remedies so that you might try them if you like. Remember that, generally, food herbal remedies are not as strong and invasive as western medicines so to see results takes more time. Those that I have chosen to translate are general remedies that can be commonly used by all. You may try them for a few months and see if you notice any changes. Remember if you have a specific health need, consult an experienced Chinese medical doctor. She or he will have the knowledge to best treat you. Also, it is important for a healthy person who wants to use food for longevity to learn more about what types of foods should not be eaten together. Certain foods can cancel each other out or can be toxic when mixed.

Spring

During the spring season, eat more light and cool-natured food, such as barley, yellow soy beans, Chinese sorghum, celery, shepherd's purse, spinach, egg plant, bamboo shoot, wax gourd, spinach gourd, carrot, cucumber, sweet melon, duck eggs, coconut, *luo han guo*, tea, liver, chicken, and Chinese dates.

Summer

During summer, your meals should be light and easy to digest, such as bread (steamed is even better) and rice and noodle soups. Other suitable foods are roasted barley flour, mung bean, spinach, lotus root, watermelon, sweet melon, melons used as vegetables, peach, lemon, coconut, sugar cane, tomato, bamboo shoot, cucumber, carrot, orange family, tofu, duck meat, grapes, and eggs. Seafood and meats that have a cool or gentle nature can also be consumed. Vinegar is beneficial.

Autumn

In autumn, foods such as *Yi yi ren* (a grain that can be find in Chinatown), Shan yao (Chinese yam), honey, peanuts, apricot seeds, white apricot, grapes, fig, lily, carrot, radish, spinach, persimmon, wax gourd seed, pear, persimmon dry fruit, mushroom, and oranges are most beneficial. You should also include foods that supply nutrition gently and have the function of moistening dryness.

Winter

In winter eat foods that are good for building yang such as: rice, wheat, black soy beans, goat spine or tail bone soup, turtle meat,

Chinese chive (*jiu tsai*), black dates, bone marrow of lamb and ox, walnut, chestnut, shrimp, lamb, and sesame seeds.

COMMON FOODS FOR LONGEVITY

The following foods are commonly consumed to help increase your life span: sesame seeds (the black kind is even better), corn, sweet yam, rice, peanut oil, peanuts, small red beans, mung beans, other beans, soy milk, tofu products (there are more varieties in Chinatown), wheat, *shan yao, Mu er* (white and black), *Xiang gu* (the dry, fragrant mushroom), green vegetables, cabbage, pumpkin seeds, sunflower seeds, carrots, apples, grapes, figs, plums, peach seeds, Chinese olives, lotus root, sesame oil, lotus seeds, lotus leaf, fish, pork kidney, heart, lung, pork feet, pork tendon, beef and tendon, chicken, duck, rabbit meat, quail meat and eggs, milk, eggs, rock sugar, lily, honey and royal jelly. When eating foods for the purpose of longevity, it is important to know what foods best complement each other so that you can get the best result possible.

COOKING

When cooking with herbs, it is better to use clay or glass cooker instead of metal.

There are many ways for cooking the above food. The most common is to boil them in water, steam them or use them in a stirfry. Generally, there are six types of stirfry. The most common way is to flavor the stirfry first with ingredients like green onion, ginger root, or pepper. Once the oil has been flavored then you can add the other ingredients.

If you are cooking with meat, it is common practice to cut it into bite sized pieces before cooking it. If you wish to tenderize it you may do so by adding a little bit of starch to it.

HERBAL WINE

Many Chinese people make herbal wine remedies at home by themselves. Such recipes can be found in Chinese cookbooks and are designed to preserve health or treat different health needs.

In preparation, make the ingredients into small pieces or powders so that they can be wrapped in a cotton cloth and placed in the wine base. This insures that the essence and not the pieces of the herbs get into the wine. The wine base can be brown as is made from sweet millet, liquor, or regular wine. The type of wine and amount used will be specified in the recipe as will the amounts and types of herbs. You will combine the herbs, wrap them in a piece of white cotton, and tie the cloth to be sure the herbs do not get out into the wine. Put the wine into a jar and place the herb bag in also. Seal the jar and set it in the corner of your kitchen, another room, or a dark or light place so that the herbal properties can be absorbed by the wine. Shake the mixture once a day for seven to ten days (the time will also be specified by the recipe). When the time is complete, remove the herb bag and the herbal wine is ready to take. The dosage and frequency will also be noted in the recipe. If you need to expedite the process the herbs and wine can be cooked together. To do this, combine ingredients in a pot and bring to a boil three times. When the mixture cools to room temperature, the wine is ready.

The most common way to prepare herbal remedies such as teas and infusions is to boil the ingredients in water. The usual practice is to boil them for half an hour and remove the liquid for use.

Following are some ancient food recipes that are still popular today. I purposely chose recipes that contain ingredients that I have seen in America so that you may try them. All these recipes are for building up good health. You will find in the appendix of this book a conversion chart from metric to American standard units.

Note. Some recipes use a clay pot. Such a pot can be purchased at little expense at a Chinese grocery store.

CANDY FOR IMPROVING MEMORY AND DARKENING HAIR

According to Chinese medicine, walnut nourishes the brain and hair; sesame seeds slow aging.

INGREDIENTS: 250 grams walnut, 250 grams black sesame seeds, 500 grams red sand sugar

PREPARATION: Grind sesame seeds and walnuts in a grinder. Dry-stirfry the sugar with a little bit of water— about 1/3 teaspoon—at a medium-high temperature until it boils. Once the mixture comes to a boil reduce the heat to low and stir mixture until it thickens. When mixture thickens add sesame seeds and walnuts, and stir the mixture until it is evenly blended. Remove the mixture from the heat and let it cool. Then place it on a cutting board and cut into date-sized chunks while it is still warm. Allow it to cool. Eat three pieces twice a day, in the morning and evening.

SESAME RICE SOUP FOR BUILDING UP BLOOD

INGREDIENTS: 30 grams black sesame, 100 grams rice

PREPARATION: Roast the sesame seeds in a pan or oven at a low temperature so that you can stir it evenly. Sesame seeds are very easily over-roasted, so be careful with the temperature and time. Grind them, then add them to the rice and cook in water. Be sure to add more water than you normally would to cook rice so that you get a soup like consistency. You can have the soup often at any time.

LONGEVITY DESSERT

INGREDIENTS: Black sesame seeds, roasted and ground, (organic) beef bone marrow, wheat flour or rice flour, enough dark sugar to add a little sweetness (amounts depending on the tastes of the individual)

PREPARATION: Place the bone marrow in a pan at a medium low temperature; as it heats you will see oil separating from the marrow. Remove the dregs from the oil.

Add the flour to the oil and stir at a medium low temperature until the flour becomes light brown.

Add the sugar and mix thoroughly to an even consistency. This mixture can then be saved in a jar in the refrigerator

To eat it, place two to three tablespoons in a bowl, and pour in some boiling water and stir into a thin gruel-like consistency. It is ready to eat.

This is a great dessert, but it is also my children's and my favorite breakfast. You can add some roasted walnuts, sesame, hazelnuts, or pecans to it if you like.

ADDING MOISTURE TO THE LUNGS AND SKIN

INGREDIENTS: 1 bone of goat (or sheep) spine chopped into big pieces, 100 grams millet, a little salt to taste.

PREPARATION: Wash and cook the bones in water until the soup is milky-white; remove the bones. Wash the millet and add to the soup and cook until done (approximately 30 minutes). Then, add the salt. Eat anytime you like.

INGREDIENTS: 500 grams sesame seeds, appropriate amount of white sugar for the taste mainly

PREPARATION: Roast the sesame seeds in an iron pan at a low temperature, then grind, and save in a jar.

When eating, get two soupspoons of the ground sesame seeds, add a little sugar to taste, and pour in hot water (half cup or less). Drink.

You can also buy roasted black sesame powder in a Chinese grocery or herb store, but make sure it is fresh.

LONGEVITY EGG FOR BUILDING UP BLOOD

Heh shou wu is a longevity herb that is sold in bottles in American markets. Egg is beneficial for building up blood. Ginger and green onion both release cold and promote qi circulation.

INGREDIENTS: 50 grams to 100 grams Heh shou wu, 2 eggs still in shells, 2 American green onions, one chunk of raw ginger root, salt to taste, cooking wine, and a little butter

PREPARATION: Wash the herb Heh shou wu clean, and cut into 3.3 cm long, 1.6 cm wide pieces. In a pan, combine all of the ingredients together, including the unbroken eggs. Add some water to barely cover the ingredients. Cook at a high temperature until boiling. Reduce heat to low and cook until the eggs are hard-boiled. Remove the eggs and soak in cold water so that the shells are easier to remove. Once the shell is removed, place the eggs back into the soup and cook for an additional two minutes. The eggs can be eaten once a day.

LOTUS SEEDS RICE SOUP FOR BUILDING UP HEALTH AND TREATING FORGETFULNESS

Memory loss usually happens to older people and is caused by bad circulation. This recipe is for building up the center of the Five Elements—the Earth—to benefit all organs.

INGREDIENTS: Fresh, tender lotus seeds 20 grams, 100 grams rice

PREPARATION: Soak the seeds until they expand, use a brush to rub off the thin skin, Remove the hearts. Place the lotus seeds in a pan and cover with water. Cook first at a high temperature until boiling, and then turn to medium-high until the seeds are mushy.

Wash the rice and cook in water until it is thin gruel; add water depending on the cook's wish: thin soup or thick. Then add in the lotus seeds, stir, and eat warm.

APRICOT SEEDS RICE SOUP FOR SOOTHING COUGH

Apricot seeds help to remove phlegm. If you do not have a cough, this soup helps build the immune system.

INGREDIENTS: 10 grams sweet, fresh apricot seeds (remove their tips and skin), 50 grams rice

PREPARATION: Grind the seeds until mushy, wash the rice, and cook them in water to make gruel.

Eat it warm, twice a day as breakfast and supper, to help sooth a cough.

PINE SEEDS RICE SOUP FOR MOISTENING THE LUNG AND FOR CONSTIPATION

Pine seeds (*Song zi*) have been a longevity food for the Chinese since ancient times. They are easy to digest, but you should only eat one tablespoon a day. Eating too much will produce heat in your body.

INGREDIENTS: 50 grams pine seeds that you can buy from organic food store or Chinatown, 50 grams rice, honey to taste

PREPARATION: Grind the seeds, and then cook them with the rice in water. When the rice is done, add a little honey to taste.

Eat on an empty stomach in the morning or before going to bed.

MULBERRY HONEY FOR LONGEVITY AND TO BUILD UP HEALTH

Mulberry tree is quite valuable and every part of it is used as an herb.

INGREDIENTS: 200 grams fresh ripe mulberries, 50 grams honey

PREPARATION: Wash the berries clean. Pound them until mushy, and separate the juice from the berry with a strainer. Place the juice in a pan and cook the juice until it thickens slightly. Add the honey and stir continuously until the mixture becomes creamy. When it is cool, save in a bottle. In the refrigerator it can last longer. Eat one to two soupspoons with warm water, twice a day in the morning and evening.

SOUP FOR WEAKNESS, ASTHMA, BUILDING UP THE KIDNEYS AND SPLEEN

It treats bronchitis, low sexual energy, or constipation.

INGREDIENTS: 60 grams rice, 80 grams deep-fried walnuts light brown in color, 45 grams raw walnuts, 200 grams (organic) cow milk, 12 grams white sand sugar

PREPARATION: Soak the rice for one hour. Grind the rice with the other ingredients in a little water and remove the liquid. Cook in water until boiling, and add the sugar. Remove dregs in the soup, and then cook again until boiling. Stir.

Eat for breakfast or as dessert.

FOR NOURISHING BLOOD, SOOTHING PREGNANCY, AND MOISTENING THE LUNGS

Er jiao is an herb made from a special donkey skin that builds up blood. (Note that the Chinese term "herb" includes any natural source that has medicinal purposes.) Sweet rice benefits the spleen.

INGREDIENTS: 15 grams Er jiao (an herb that you get from a Chinese herbal store), 100 grams sweet rice.

PREPARATION: Cook the rice into soup first, then break Er jiao into pieces and add it the soup. It will melt.

Eat it warm, twice a day in the morning and at supper.

LONGEVITY SHAN YAO RICE SOUP

Shan yao is a longevity food. The dried kind works best.

INGREDIENTS: 30 grams dry Shan yao (Chinese yam, get from Chinese grocery or herbal store), 50 grams sweet rice

PREPARATION: Cook together into soup with a little sugar. This is good for all the seasons. Eat it warm.

FOR YIN DEFICIENCY SYNDROMES, ALSO HELPS PROMOTE BREAST MILK

INGREDIENTS: 45 grams raw peanuts with skin, 30 grams Shan yao, 100 grams rice, appropriate amount of rock sugar to bring to taste.

PREPARATION: Grind peanuts and Shan yao in a grinder, and cook with rice into gruel. When done, add the sugar.

Eat this as a meal once or twice a day.

FOR NOURISHING THE BLOOD AND MOISTENING DRYNESS

INGREDIENTS: 250 grams spinach, 250 grams rice, appropriate amount of salt to add flavor

PREPARATION: Wash the spinach clean. Dip in boiling water and take them out at once. Cut into small pieces. Wash the rice and boil in water to make soup. When the rice soup is done, add in spinach and salt to taste.

Eat it as a meal as often as you wish.

INGREDIENTS: 10 grams white ginseng, 10 dried lotus seeds, 30 grams rock sugar

PREPARATION: Soak ginseng and the seeds together in water until they expanded. Add the sugar, put in a steamer, and steam for one hour.

Drink the soup and eat the seeds once a day, as long as you need. The ginseng can be reused the same way three times. The third time, you can eat the ginseng.

GINSENG RICE SOUP FOR BUILDING UP THE ORGANS

Caution: do not eat ginseng with radish or tea, and do not eat in a hot season; it is not for people who have yin deficiency and strong fire or for strong, healthy individuals.

INGREDIENTS: 3 grams ginseng powder (or 15 grams Dang shen powder as substitute), 60 grams rice, a little rock sugar to taste

PREPARATION: Combine ingredients and cook them in a clay pot in water until done. This is good to eat on an empty stomach in the morning, in autumn and winter.

FOR NOURISHING THE SPLEEN AND HEART

Lotus seed is named the "spleen-fruit." It is good to cook it with grains, pork, and many other tonic herbs. *Bai he* (lily root) is especially good for women. It balances emotions and nourishes the organs. Pork has gentle nature, and functions similar to lotus and Bai he. Both of the herbs can be found in a Chinese grocery store.

INGREDIENTS: 50 grams lotus seeds, 50 grams Bai he, 250 grams sliced pork

PREPARATION: Cook them in clay pot in water on the top of stove. When soup is boiling, add some green onion and salt; turn to lower temperature to simmer the soup until done. Drink and eat as long as you wish.

FOR TREATING FORGETFULNESS AND SOOTHING THE LUNGS AND HEART

Bai he-Yin er Soup
Yin er is a dried white mushroom that you can only get in Chinatown. It builds up the kidneys and benefits the lungs.

INGREDIENTS: 50 grams Bai he, 50 grams lotus seeds, 25 grams Yin er

PREPARATION: Soak Yin er in warm water to clean and remove the hard "bud." Combine the Bai he and lotus seeds in water, and bring to a boil. Add Yin er. Cook them at a low temperature, and add some rock sugar to taste. Cook until the soup thickens.

LONGEVITY FORMULA

The leaves of cypress are one of the longevity herbs.

INGREDIENTS: Cypress leaves. Pick the leaves in any season, chop them fine, and steam them in a sealed bottle for several hours. Remove the leaves, and shower them with boiling then cold water repeatedly. Dry in the shade until they are completely dried. Make them into powder and take 20 grams with warm water before a meal, twice a day.

FOR PEOPLE WHO DO MENTAL WORK

Herbs like royal jelly, honey, flower pollens, and chrysanthemum flowers, are good for people who do mental work. You can get the ingredients in the following recipe from a Chinese herbal store.

INGREDIENTS: Equal amount of *Jin yin* flowers, *Mai men dong*, chrysanthemum flowers, black sesame seeds, *Yuan zhi* powder, *Shan zha* (chopped), *Gan cao* (*tsao*) powder.

PREPARATION: Combine the ingredients and grind into a powder. When making a drink, use 3–5 teaspoon of mixture, 0.5 teaspoon of honey, 0.5 teaspoon of flower pollen, and pour in about one cup of water. Eat it warm daily, once a day.

GENERAL ACTION OF SOME FOODS

❖ Foods such as liver, egg, beans, shrimp, sesame seeds, and celery leaves are known to build up the blood.

❖ Fresh vegetables aid in the removal of toxins found in our cells. Such toxins are filtered by the kidneys and excreted out in the urine.

❖ Mung bean has the nature to releases various kinds of poisons which have been proven in thousands years of Chinese life experience. Many herbal formulas are not taken with this mung bean soup because it can reduce the herb's function.

❖ Mushrooms are very good at cleansing toxins in the blood.

❖ Tofu made with pig blood, called *Zhu xie to fu,* cleanses most toxins in human blood. It can be cooked as a stirfry with other vegetables.

The material provided above is only the tip of the iceberg when it comes to herbal and food cures. I wanted to wet you appetite, so to speak, so that you would see how these remedies are integrated into our daily lives. All that we have discussed is part of the cultivation process, and all aspects of this cultivation process are meant to make you more balanced mentally, physically, and emotionally.

TRANSLATIONS

"Tips for cooking"
— Gao Lian

To cook fresh water fish, boiling the water first then put in the fish, the fish bone will be crispy.

To cook fish from the ocean and big river, boiling the source [ocean or big river water] first, then put in the fish, the fish bone will be firm (and will be easier to remove).

By adding in a couple of bases of persimmons when cooking, the color of the crab will retain the same.

To make dried shrimp,* dry-stirfry them in salt and rinse off the salt. Their color will remain naturally red.

To preserve tangerine family, use pine leaves to wrap. In this way, for three to four months their freshness will remain.

For tender taste vegetable, dipping the greens in boiling water and then quickly get them into cold water. To make this vegetable a salad or to dry it, its color and tenderness will be preserved.

To cook meat, avoid using the wood of a mulberry tree.

To correct the wine that becomes sour, put a cotton bag in the wine, which contains one liter of small red beans that have been roasted light brown (crispy). Then the wine will turn out fine.

To clean a fish, drop a few drops of uncooked oil on it. The sticky fluid will be removed.

For better tasting meat and done quicker, just add some fruit of paper mulberry tree, and cook with the lid on.

To cook goose meat faster, add a few leaves of the peach tree.

*Dried shrimp can be a "spice" to add flavor in Chinese cooking or can be cooked as a dish. You can find them Chinatown.

"The Five-spice-sour Dressing"
- Gao Lian

INGREDIENTS:
1 soup spoon of salted fermented soy bean sauce, 0.18oz dark vinegar, 0.18oz white sugar, 5–7 Chinese pepper seeds' shells (hua jiao), 2 black pepper seeds, 1 piece of fresh ginger root, 2 garlic cloves.
Grind the seeds and blend the rest together."

References

Ancient

I Ching, Author unknown

Tao De Jing, Lao Ji (Li Ren)

Ben Cao (aka *Shen Nong Ben Cao, Herbal Classic*) Shen Nong

The Yellow Emperor's Internal Classic, Author unknown

Lei Classic (Classified Canon), Zhang Jie-bin

The Eight Fields of Preserving Your Life with Respect, Gao Lian (Ming Dynasty)

Gynecology and Obstetrics, Fu Qing-zhu

The Causes of Diseases, Chao Yuan-fang

The Complete Effective Prescription for Women's Diseases, Chen Zi-ming

Materia Medica, Li Shi-Zhen

Contemporary

The Definitions of Zhou I by the Ancient Famous Physician, Heh Shao-chu

Probe Qigong, Tao Bin-fu

Index

BOOKS & VIDEOS FROM YMAA

YMAA Publication Center Books

YMAA Publication Center Videotapes

YMAA PUBLICATION CENTER 楊氏東方文化出版中心

4354 Washington Street Roslindale, MA 02131
1-800-669-8892 • ymaa@aol.com • www.ymaa.com